The Accidental Farmer's Blueberry Cookbook

....

People might forget what you said.
But they'll never forget what you fed them.
Ann Handley

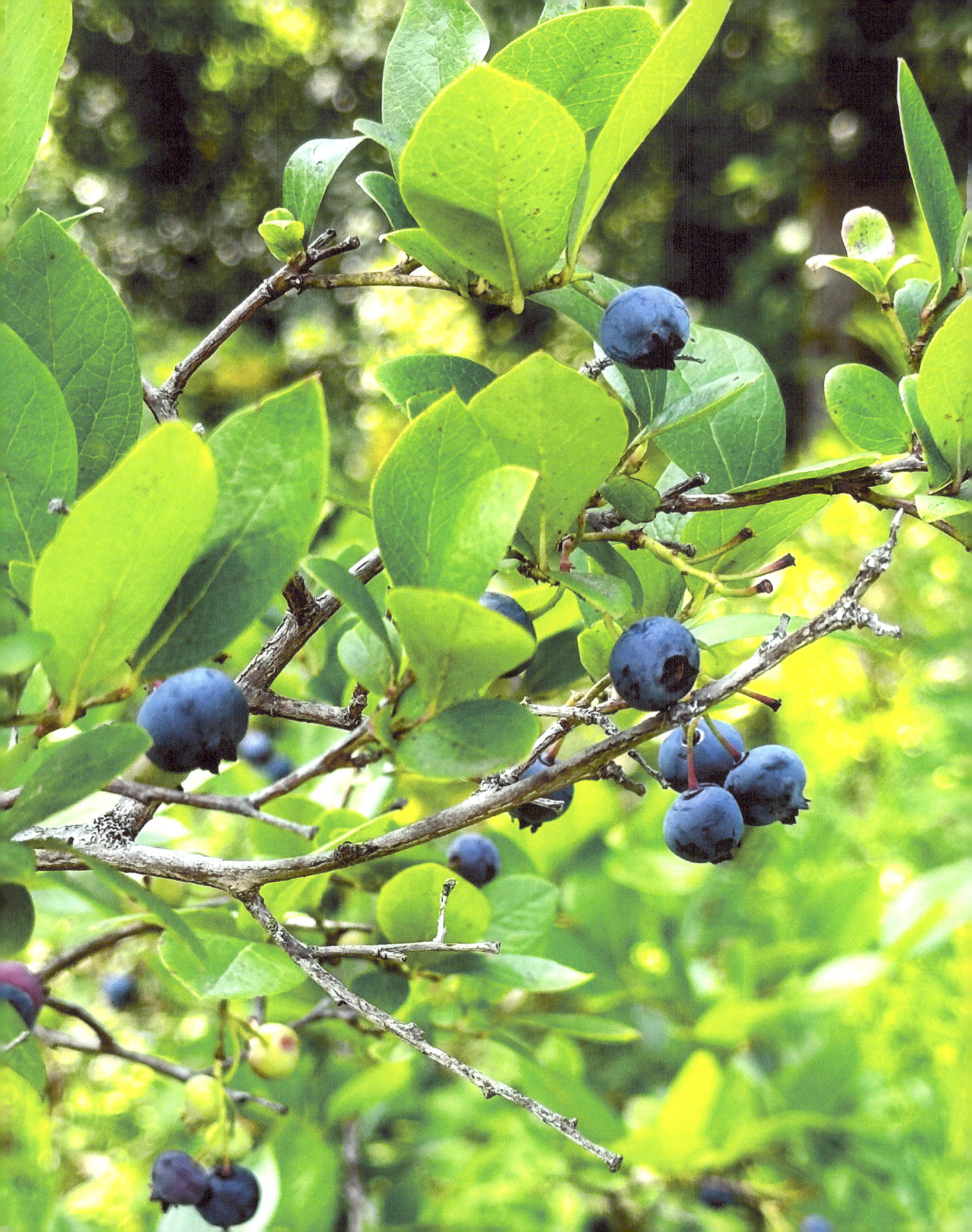

The Accidental Farmer's Blueberry Cookbook

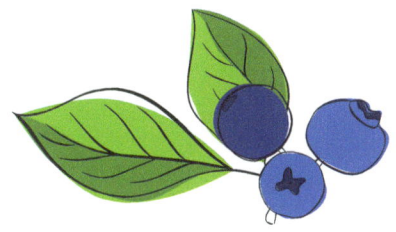

SWEET & SAVORY RECIPE COLLECTIONS
FOR YEAR-ROUND COOKING

Dorothy Stainbrook
(from FarmtoJar.com)

Copyright © 2025 by Dorothy Stainbrook

All rights reserved. No part of this publication may be reproduced, stored in a retrieval system, or transmitted in any form or by any means—electronic, mechanical, photocopying, recording, or otherwise—without the prior written permission of Dorothy Stainbrook, except in the case of brief quotations used in critical articles or reviews.

This book is intended for informational purposes only. The author and publisher are not responsible for any adverse effects or consequences resulting from the use of the recipes or suggestions contained in this book. Always consult your physician or a qualified health provider before making dietary changes, especially if you have food allergies or medical conditions.

Paperback ISBN: 979-8-9924630-3-3

Hardcover ISBN: 979-8-9924630-5-7

Photography by: Dorothy Stainbrook

iStock Images:
Aleksei Bezrukov p.135; Al Gonzalez p.101, 162; Artit Wongpradu p.145; Ekaterina Lektorskaia p.38; manyakotic p.41; Nazar Nazaruk p.13; Stephanie Frey p.157; tenkende p.21

Illustrations by: Jane Heldman & Dorothy Stainbrook

Book Design by: Molly Seabrook, Credible Ink

Independently Published

For more information, visit: Dorothy Stainbrook: From Farm to Jar (FarmtoJar.com)

Printed in the United States of America

First edition

DEDICATION

For my daughter, who is an ongoing inspiration of courage and possibilities, and for my son, the most competitive blueberry picker imaginable in this girly profession.

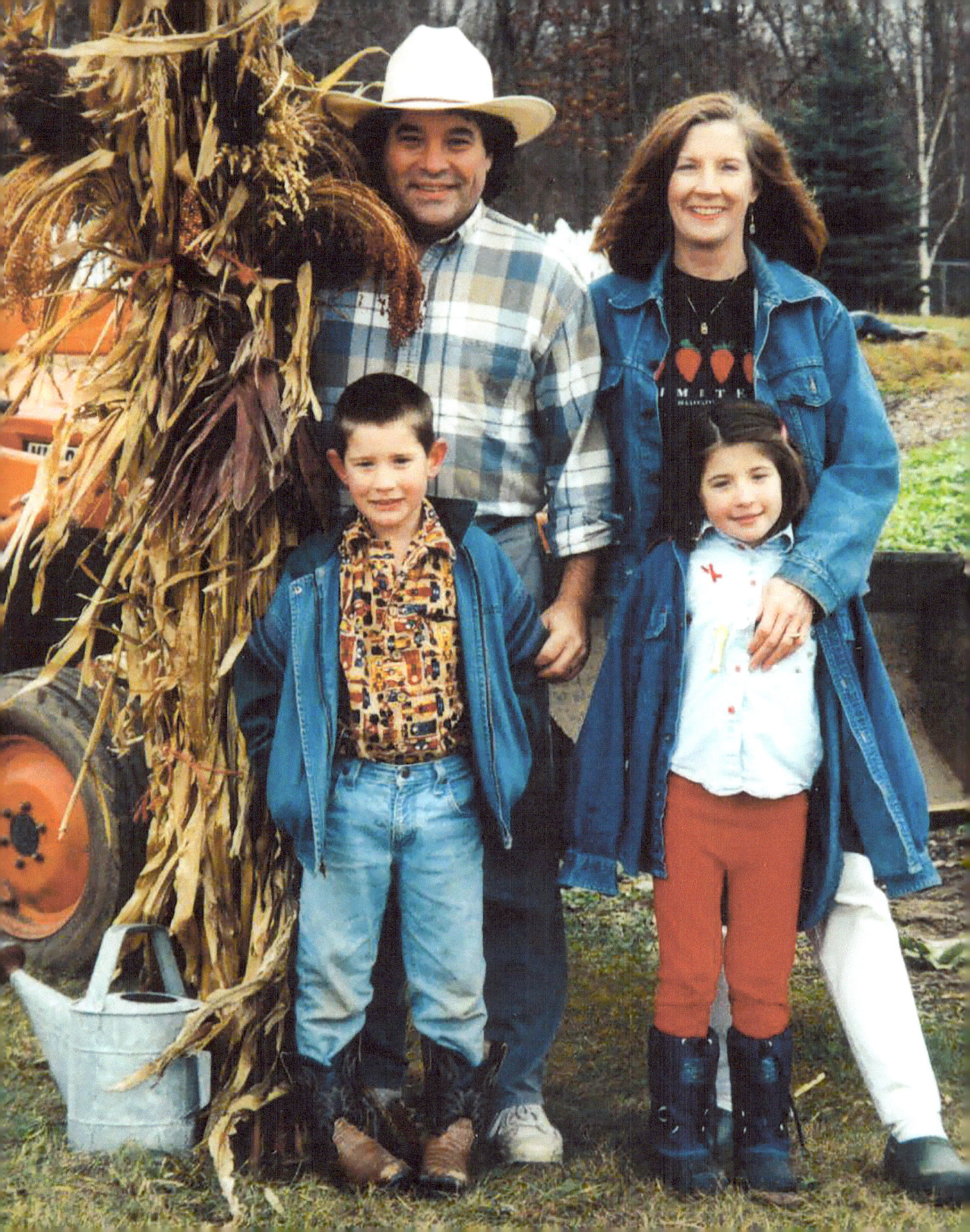

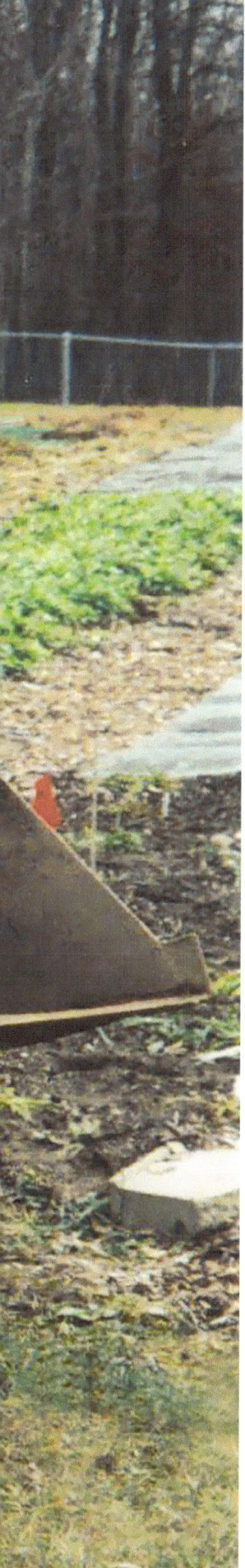

The Accidental Farmer: From Heartbreak To Harvest

Thank you for checking out my blueberry cookbook! My journey to becoming a farmer and accomplished home cook came about quite unexpectedly—hence the name "Accidental Farmer".

I certainly didn't start out loving to cook. And as for farming—my first experience was buying a root-bound 6-pack of tomatoes, planting them as a whole pack in our lawn, and watching them die, lol. Growing blueberries? Well, that was a whole different ballgame that was totally out of my league.

Everything changed when my daughter was born. She was born with only one working ventricle in her heart and was going to require indefinite hands-on care.

My husband and I assessed our financial situation and decided it would make more sense for me to quit my job and provide the hands-on care she needed rather than him, as his salary was higher. We knew we'd need every penny for what lay ahead.

As our little family progressed on this new, unknown path, I found I needed a creative outlet to explore as I tended to my daughter's various surgeries and health issues. We happened to live on 23 acres of weed-infested land, so I decided to roll up my sleeves and become a farmer! Why not? Couldn't be that hard, right?

Over time, I did learn how to grow tomatoes from seed rather than a sad 6-pack, and I planted and tended 600 organic blueberry plants. It was the blueberries that truly captured my heart though. These remarkable little berries seemed to embody everything I was learning about resilience, patience, and the sweet rewards that come from nurturing something with care.

Six years into this new adventure, I knew I had earned my farmer credentials when I had the classic conversation with my young son about what he wanted to be when he grew up. After posing the question, he went into deep thought mode. I finally suggested, "Would you want to be a farmer?" He looked at me incredulously and said, "No way! That's a girl's job".

Over the next 15 years, the kids and I sold blueberries and heirloom tomatoes at the larger farmers' markets in the Twin Cities. I was so grateful that I was able to provide my two children with a beautiful, enchanted childhood on our little farm.

My daughter was able to grow up with a parent at her side, and although she is not cured, she is leading a very productive life as a school social worker in the Denver metro area.

My son learned high finance and people skills by selling with me at the markets. He's very competitive and became not only the fastest blueberry picker, but also highly skilled at communicating with people of all ages and backgrounds. Guess what field he went into? It's no surprise to me that he chose a career in finance and is doing well these days at at a Colorado investment firm.

As for myself, I never returned to a corporate job, but over time my focus shifted, pivoting in a number of directions that all started with the farm. We converted our garage into a commercial kitchen where I turned all of those luscious blueberries into preserves for the market. The commercial kitchen also functioned as a place to develop and test recipes for my food blog.

Today I share my experiences with food, diet and gardening on my website, "Farm to Jar", as well as in a weekly newsletter, and now books. My first book focused on growing heirloom tomatoes. This second book, however, shares blueberry-forward recipes sprinkled with my experiences raising kids and dogs on a rural plot of land in Central Minnesota.

Oh, and I visit both kids in Colorado every chance I get. Neither one of them wanted to take on that "girly" work of farming!

Yours truly,
The Accidental Farmer

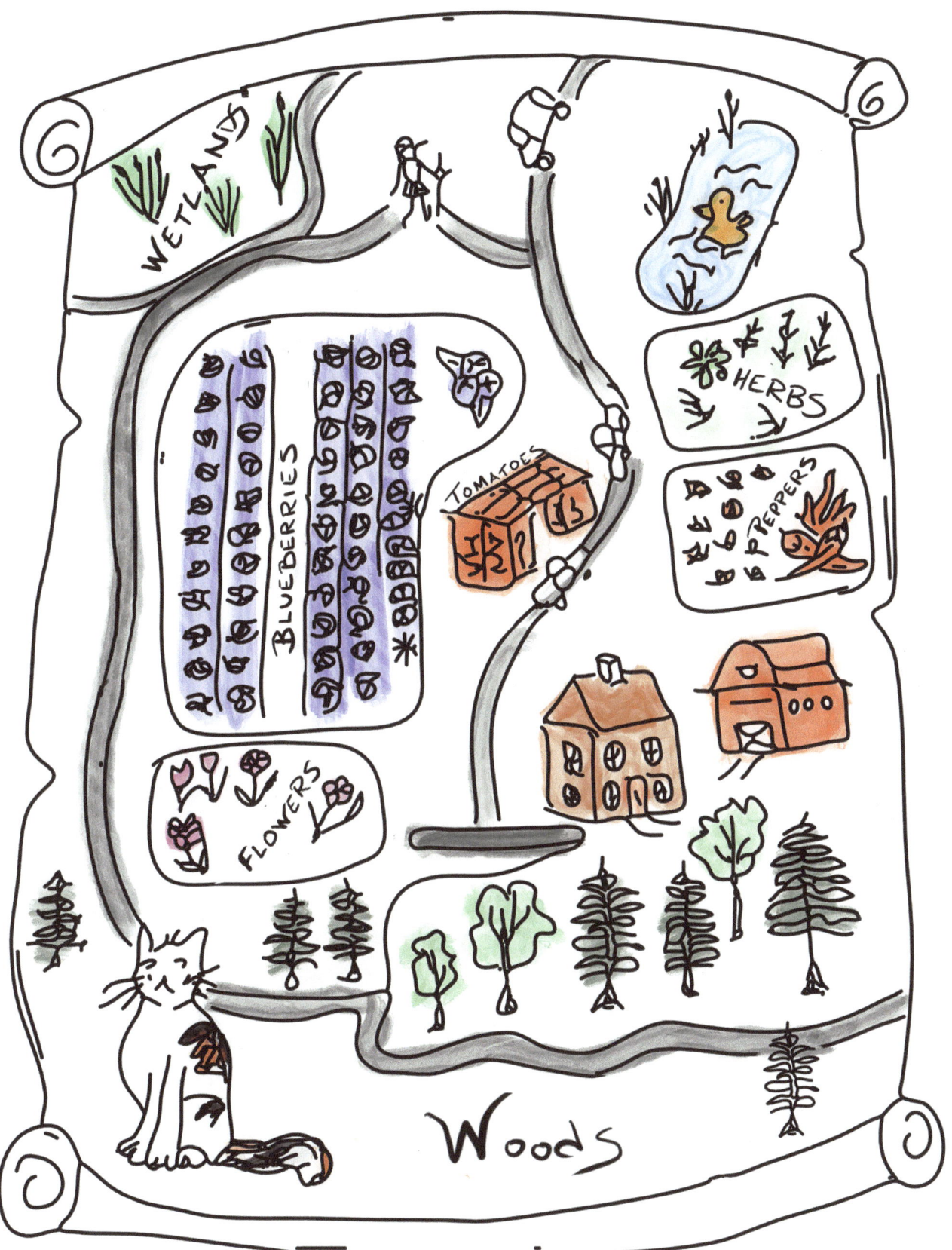

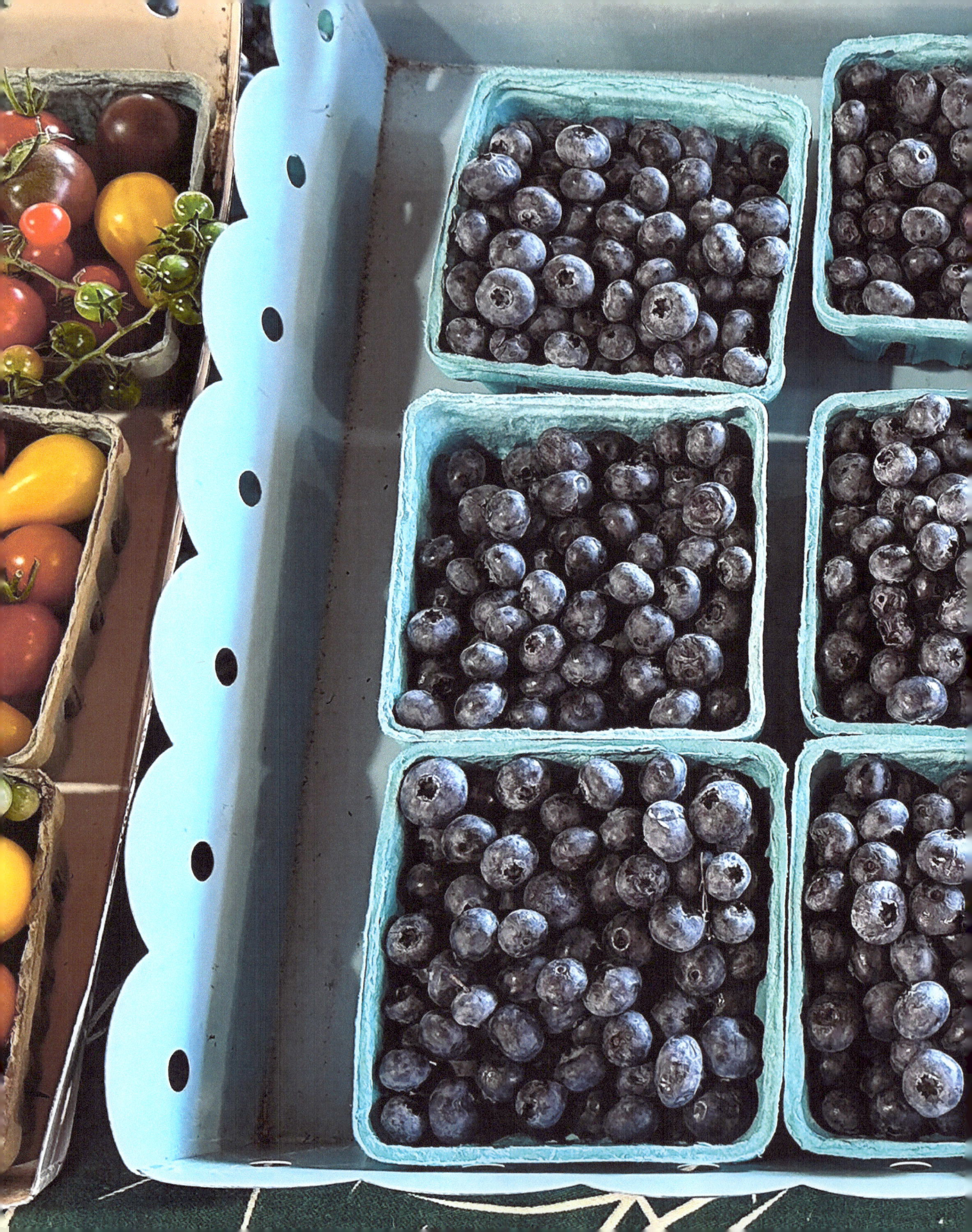

TABLE OF CONTENTS

Part I - Getting Started

How to Use this Cookbook 2
A Useful Pantry 4
Tools & Equipment 9
Blueberries 101 13

Part II - Let's Cook

BREAKFAST 19
SAVORY MAIN DISHES 49
EASY RUSTIC DESSERTS 67
SUNDAY DESSERT PROJECTS 91
DRINKS 113
CONDIMENTS & PRESERVES 127
FOUNDATIONAL RECIPES 145

Part III - Helpful Resources

Links for Further Information 161
Conversion Chart 175
Index 163
Acknowledgments 167
About the Author 169

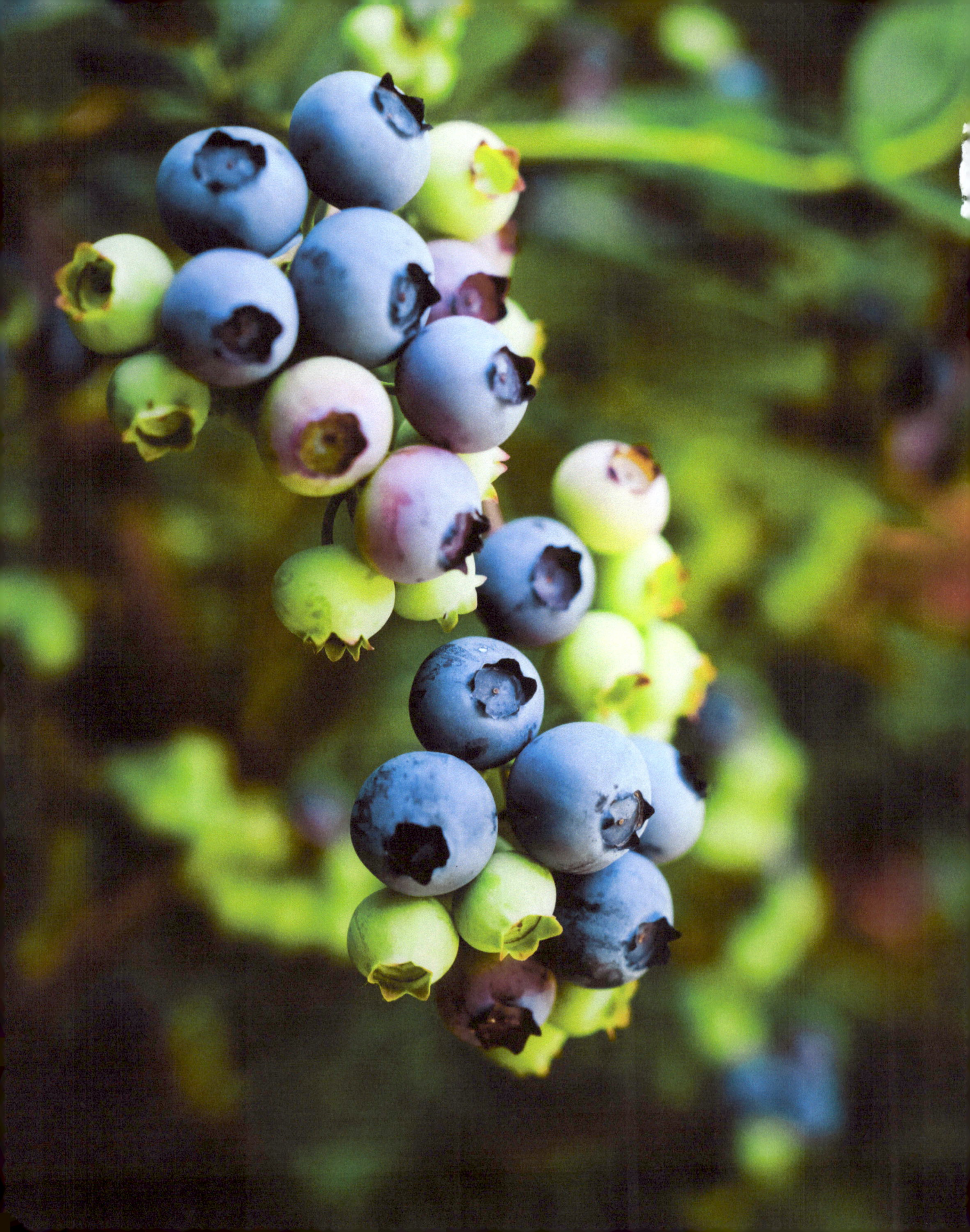

Part I
Getting Started

How to Use This Book

MY COOKING PHILOSOPHY

I was a slow-carb diet coach back when Tim Ferriss's 4-Hour Body diet was popular. I actually saw a lot of success with fat loss on that diet, both for myself and over 400 clients.

One of the tenets of the diet that kept it sustainable was the idea of a "Cheat Day". One client said it felt like Christmas once a week. This form of delayed gratification was maligned by many, and I wouldn't vouch for cheat day in terms of health, but I will say it was quite effective for fat loss.

The slow-carb diet taught me to truly savor the full flavor of desserts; they were truly treats rather than a daily occurrence.

So, in developing the recipes in this book, the main priority was to highlight the flavor of the berries, while taking it easy on the sugar.

Additionally, as a recipe developer and writer, my aim is to share what I have learned in a way that is both inspirational and clear to a home cook, whether beginner or advanced.

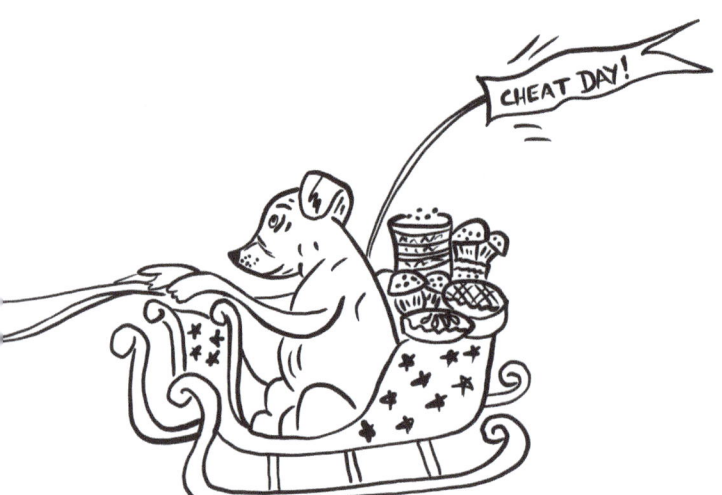

Here are a few details that will help while using these recipes:

Scratch vs store-bought

I use high-quality store-bought ingredients when they will not take away from flavor, but will save time (e.g., the flatbread pizza or the ice cream sandwiches). If something is critical to the flavor or texture of the final dish, I will provide the "from scratch" recipe (e.g., the blueberry pie).

Baking times vs "or until"

All ovens are different, so I will note the time it took in my oven so you have a general idea, but I also add an "or until" comment as a doneness indicator. For example, "bake at 400°F for 20 minutes, or until the edges are golden brown and a toothpick comes out clean".

Serving size vs size of baking dish

This is tricky. A serving for my 30-year-old son is going to be different from a serving for grandma. I will therefore note the size of the pan it was cooked in and estimate the number of typical servings so that I can calculate an accurate nutrition analysis.

Easy-to-Difficult Ratings

The difficulty rating is noted at the top of the recipe with 1-3 whisk icons, signifying easy, medium, or difficult. The ratings are subjective and based on the comments from my home cook recipe testers.

Substitutions & Additions

I'm not well-versed in gluten-free or non-dairy cooking, so many of my substitutions do not address the type of flour or dairy that can be successfully substituted. I leave it to you to know how to change a recipe to meet any specific diet restrictions. I do, however, include a number of variations that have been tested by either myself or the recipe testers.

Cooking Notes

I will note when certain techniques or ingredients are important to the success of the recipe. While most of my recipes are fairly easy, some recipes require attention to detail.

Nutrition (Macros vs. Overwhelm)

As noted in my above philosophy, I was a low-carb diet coach for a number of years, and I found that for most people, the calorie count, the macros, and the sugar are the critical things to track for health and/or weight loss. For the sake of space, therefore, I do not include all of the micronutrient information.

Grams vs. Cups vs. Ounces vs. Milliliters
BLUEBERRIES

For blueberries in particular, the weight of a pint or a cup will most always vary. Some blueberries are small and dense but take up less room, and sometimes you will be using frozen blueberries instead of fresh.

- The good thing here is that it doesn't really impact the success of the recipe if the amount of blueberries is not a perfectly standardized weight.
- I use a default weight of ounces rather than grams, with 1 cup of blueberries equal to approximately 6 ounces. If you want to use the metric system, 1 cup of blueberries is about 190 grams, but it will vary based on the type of blueberry.

FLOUR, SUGAR, & DRY BULK INGREDIENTS

For flour, sugar and dry bulk ingredients, accuracy can be critical to the recipe's success in terms of structure and texture. In this case, I have provided measurements in cups for American bakers, but also in grams for those who use the metric system. Weighing the dry ingredients is by far the most accurate option and is more important in baking than in other types of cooking.

BUTTER

Butter is measured in tablespoons and in grams.

DRY INGREDIENTS

Small amounts of dry ingredients like salt, baking powder, baking soda, etc. are measured in teaspoons and/or tablespoons, and I do not list the gram weight.

LIQUID INGREDIENTS

Liquid ingredients are measured by volume rather than weight. I have noted liquid measurements both in cups and milliliters.

Note: A metric equivalent chart is provided in the back of this cookbook to help with conversions.

A Useful Pantry

The basic building blocks needed for the recipes in this book include flour, butter, sugar, eggs and salt. Oh, and of course blueberries!

To get the best results from these recipes, use ingredients that are as close to those listed in the recipe as possible. Tested substitutions are noted in each recipe. I would encourage you to modify and experiment, but with the understanding that the end result may not look or taste exactly the same as the original recipe.

Here are the useful ingredients I keep on hand, and the reasoning behind each one:

Flour

All of the recipes in this book were made with Gold Medal all-purpose flour. Many people these days follow a gluten-free diet and there is a huge range of different flours that can be used in baking. I am not well-versed in gluten-free flours, and I don't know how different flours will affect the texture of the final product, so I stick with all-purpose flour. I'm sure many gluten-free substitutions can be successful, but all of the recipes in this particular book have only been tested with all-purpose flour.

Cornmeal

I use a fine yellow cornmeal for baking, as it hydrates easily and is a nice golden color. Coarse cornmeal would be more appropriate for things like polenta, but I find a fine-grained cornmeal better for baked goods.

Oats (instant vs rolled vs steel cut)

Instant, rolled, and steel-cut oats are processed in different ways, which will affect the cooking time, texture and flavor of the recipe.

Instant oats are pre-cooked and rolled thin. They can become quite mushy when used in recipes. I don't use instant oats in any of my recipes.

Rolled oats are steamed and flattened into flakes and will hold their shape well during cooking. I used these oats in the recipes that included toppings like crumbles or crisps.

Steel cut oats are chewier and firmer than rolled or instant oats and they take longer to cook. The nutty flavor comes through more with steel cut oats. I used them in the overnight oats recipe.

Sugar

Granulated white sugar: If the recipe does not specify a certain kind of sugar, but rather just lists sugar in the ingredient list, I am referring to granulated white sugar. It is relevant to note that cutting back on the sugar may result in problems (collapsing cakes, weeping pies, cookies that don't

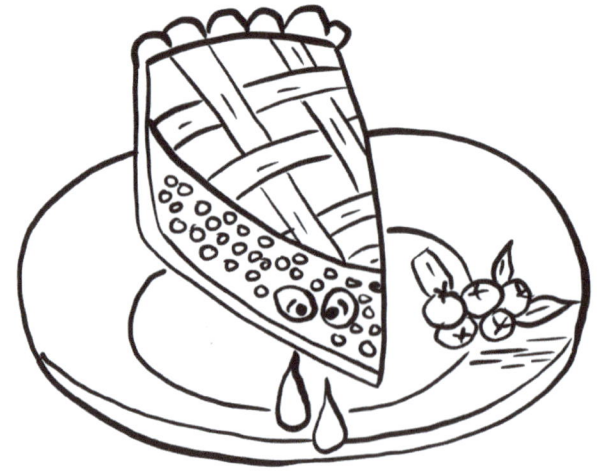

spread or brown properly, etc.). Most of my recipes err on the less sweet side of things (remnants from when I was a diet coach), but they have been tested to work.

Powdered sugar: The ultra-fine texture of powdered sugar (aka confectioner's sugar) is used for making smooth frostings, icings and glazes, as it dissolves easily. It is also great to sift on top of a dessert just before serving for visual appeal.

Brown sugar: I like to use light brown sugar rather than dark brown sugar because it allows the natural browning of cookies and cakes to come through. Light brown sugar has only 10% added molasses and is therefore milder in flavor than dark brown sugar.

Turbinado or Demerara sugar: These raw cane sugars have larger crystals and are used primarily as garnishes or finishing sugars on top of the batter before baking to add a crunch and a touch of extra sweetness.

Salt

Salt goes a long way in enhancing flavor. Making these recipes without salt may leave them bland and wanting flavor. Consumers have been bombarded with the message that salt is bad for your health, but that is not accurate when it comes to home cooking. While it is true that processed food tends to have an unhealthy amount of salt, it is rare that home-cooked food is over-salted.

The recipes in this cookbook are made with Diamond Crystal kosher salt, as it is a 100-percent pure salt. Different brands of kosher salt have different densities, but if you want to replace Diamond Crystal kosher salt with a fine-grained salt, use half the amount called for in the recipe.

Butter

All of my recipes were developed with unsalted butter so that the cook can add the level of salt to their personal preference. I use primarily Kerrygold unsalted butter, but many of the testers used a range of readily available unsalted butter brands with good results.

The main thing to pay attention to in the recipe is if it calls for room temperature butter or chilled butter. That can be a game-changer. If the recipe calls for room temperature or softened butter, let it sit out on the counter for at least two hours beforehand. Avoid microwaving butter as melted butter will behave differently. If the recipe calls for chilled butter, it means straight from the fridge.

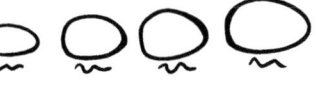

Eggs

My recipes call for eggs by number rather than by weight. The weight differences between medium sized eggs and large eggs is minor, but the difference between small and extra large eggs is significant. I use large eggs in all of the recipes. Probably best to avoid extra large eggs or small eggs—opt for medium or large and you should be fine.

When a recipe calls for eggs to be separated, keep in mind that it's easiest to do so when the eggs are cold because the yolk is more firm.

If a recipe calls for room temperature eggs but you don't have time to let them come to room temperature on the counter, place them in a bowl of hot water for a few minutes.

Blueberries

Probably 80% of the recipes in this book were made with slightly thawed frozen blueberries. I happened to have a freezer full and handed out frozen berries to all of the testers that were local. I did not find it necessary to flour the frozen berries as some recipes tell you to. I did find that there was far less bleeding using frozen berries in the baked goods as opposed to fresh.

There are some recipes where fresh berries are preferable however (such as the chicken dinner salad or the overnight oatmeal). I noted whether to use fresh or frozen when it made a difference in taste or texture.

Several of the recipes use dried blueberries (such as Earl Grey Tea Scones or Blueberry Looseleaf Tea). When I use dried blueberries in a recipe, I am using berries that are dried to the point where their texture is similar to craisins, rather than the freeze dried berries that are bone dry. Freeze dried berries shatter into tiny bits and are more useful as a topping or a powder rather than an ingredient you fold into a muffin or scone.

Lavender

Just make sure you use culinary lavender rather than the lavender used for potpourri. Look for dried culinary lavender in health food stores, or order online. I get mine in bulk from San Francisco Herb Company.

Milk

Most of the recipes in this book call for whole milk, and substituting in 2% or skim milk will change the nature of the dish, sometimes dramatically.

Some recipes, like puddings, will require whole milk for the perfect texture and flavor. It is not quite as critical in recipes that use a lot of butter, like cookies and cakes. Whole milk contains 3.5 to 4% fat, and because fat is a tenderizer, the texture of your baked good will often have a better "mouthfeel" when using whole milk.

I do list substitutions that work in some cases (such as heavy cream or sour cream). If it is not mentioned in the substitutions, change the milk at your own peril.

Thickeners:
Tapioca Powder vs Cornstarch vs Flour

Tapioca powder is my favorite thickening agent for fruit pies, as it is light rather than thick and gelatinous. It is important to note that you need to use tapioca powder (aka tapioca starch) rather than instant tapioca, and it is not always easy to find. Look for it in the gluten-free areas of your grocery store. The general recommendation is to substitute 1 tablespoon of cornstarch with 2 tablespoons of tapioca powder.

Cornstarch is widely available and gives a shiny translucent filling to pies. It gives a firmer texture in baked goods, and is commonly used in sauces and puddings.

Cornstarch can be affected by acidic ingredients however, and blueberry recipes are frequently paired with lemon zest and lemon juice, so if you can find tapioca powder it would be a preferable thickener with recipes that have a lot of lemon juice.

Flour is a standard thickener, but it is my least favorite thickener. It can make fillings appear cloudy and I can always taste it in the filling. It also requires more of it to achieve the same level of thickening as tapioca powder or cornstarch.

Leavening agents:
Baking Soda vs Baking Powder

No matter how many times I read about these two ingredients, I would always confuse them. Finally I stumbled on this saying: "Powder for the puff, and soda for the spread". While there is much more to it than that, this little saying helped me remember when to use baking powder when I didn't have time to look it up (again). They do react differently depending on the acidity of the recipe, however, and cannot be substituted for each other.

BAKING POWDER

Baking powder is added to baked goods that require a lift (hence the powder=puff), and a light open texture.

Baking soda is used with recipes that contain an acidic ingredient like lemon juice, sour cream or yogurt. Baking soda also helps with browning, adding a more complex flavor.

Sour Cream vs Cream Cheese vs Ricotta vs Yogurt

In baked goods, these four dairy products are often used interchangeably, but each of them does offer unique contributions to flavor and texture.

Sour cream adds a tangy flavor and moisture, resulting in a tender baked good or a soft crumb;

Cream cheese provides a richer, creamier flavor and texture, and is often used in frostings;

Ricotta is softer and less dense than cream cheese, with a mild flavor. It is known for preventing baked goods from drying out;

Yogurt adds a tangy, slightly sweet flavor to baked goods, and can be used when you want a lower fat alternative. Regular yogurt is not a good substitute for Greek yogurt, however, due to the different moisture contents.

Vanilla

I use Molina Mexican Vanilla Blend, simply because I like the taste and it is affordable. If you shop online you can get some quality vanilla for much less than what you pay in the supermarket. Try to avoid imitation vanilla, as it is often full of fillers and has little flavor.

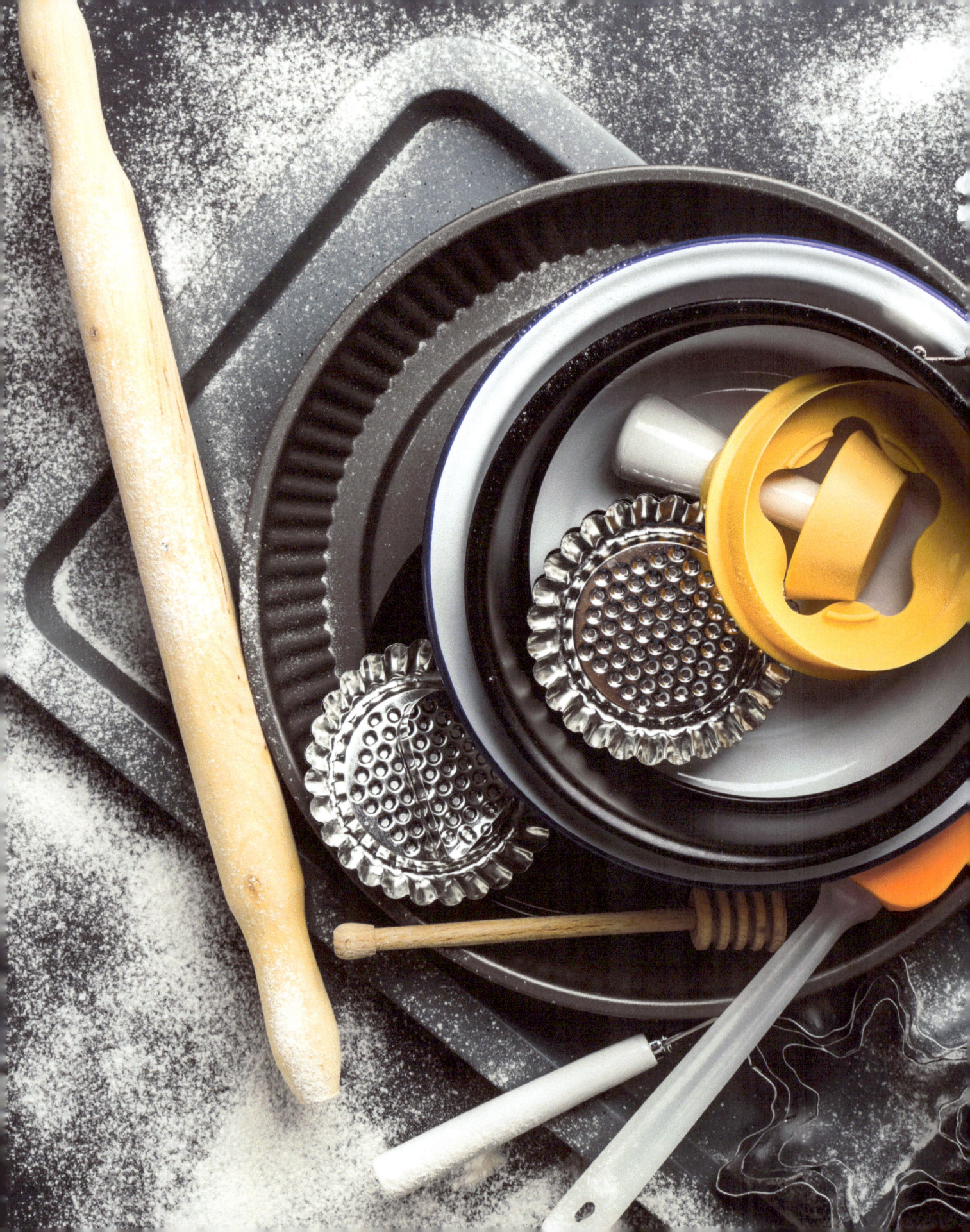

Tools & Equipment

I'm not big on specialty tools that take up a lot of counter space and are only used occasionally. That said, there are some tools that are quite helpful if you like to bake. The following tools are the ones I used to make the recipes in this book:

BAKING DISHES

Size

I do note in the recipe the size of baking dish I used, but sometimes you will just need to use what you have on hand. Most of the time the size and shape won't matter a great deal, especially with the rustic desserts. It may, however, result in a thicker or thinner baked good than you wanted, and you may have to adjust cooking times. See the chart at the end of this section for baking dish equivalents.

Metal vs Glass vs Non-Stick

A heavy-duty, light-colored, anodized aluminum baking pan is optimal. These metal pans allow more consistency throughout the baked good, as they heat and cool quickly and evenly.

Glass baking pans are great for fruit pies, allowing you to see the browning around the sides and bottom. For cakes, however, the glass remains hot after removing from the oven, which can dry out the baked goods..

Non-stick pans have a coating that may flake off with heavy use and many cooks find that unhealthy.

Cookie sheets (aka sheet pans) should be light-colored to help prevent cookies from browning too much. Non-stick sheet pans are not recommended, as they are usually black, and darker pans may result in burning along the sides.

Muffin tins are usually made of metal, but you can also find them in stoneware and silicone. Stoneware doesn't brown the muffins as well as metal, and silicone tins need to be set on a sheet pan before being put into the oven.

SPECIALTY BAKEWARE

Crêpe Pans

A pan with no side rims is needed for making crêpes. The pan should be either cast iron, heavy aluminum, or carbon steel, as these metals will heat up evenly. If you make a lot of crêpes, a specially crêpe pan is truly useful.

I used an 8-inch crêpe pan with a little wooden spreader for the recipes, but I have also used my cast iron comal with success.

Removable Bottom Tart Pan

Tart pans come in different shapes—round, square, or rectangular. They have a removable bottom so that you can remove the tart from the pan without destroying the crust. They are usually shallow with a higher crust-to-filling ratio, as the fillings tend to be quite rich. I used a tart pan in the blueberry sour cream pie, as it was difficult to remove from a regular pie pan.

SPECIALTY BAKEWARE (cont.)

8-, 10-, and 12-inch skillets, ovenproof

¾ cup (about 6 oz) ramekins for individual desserts like pudding soufflé

Metal loaf pan (4½ by 8½ inches) for the semifreddo

USEFUL SMALL TOOLS

Microplane for zesting lemons

Heatproof flexible spatulas

Digital kitchen scale

Dry measuring cups & spoons

Liquid measuring cups (1-, 2-, and 4-cup)

Fine mesh sieve

Mixing bowls (small, medium and large)

Rolling pin

Tongs

Parchment paper

Wire whisks (stainless steel)

Potato masher (for blueberry compotes)

Good oven mitts

1-ounce and 2-ounce spring-loaded scoops

Small and medium saucepans

Cooling racks

Your hands!!

USEFUL SMALL APPLIANCES

Blender (Vitamix is most powerful)

Immersion Blender
(as alternative to Vitamix)

Stand Mixers
(best for whipped cream & creaming batters)

Electric Hand Mixers
(easier to move around in the bowl)

Electric juicer (for juicing lemons)

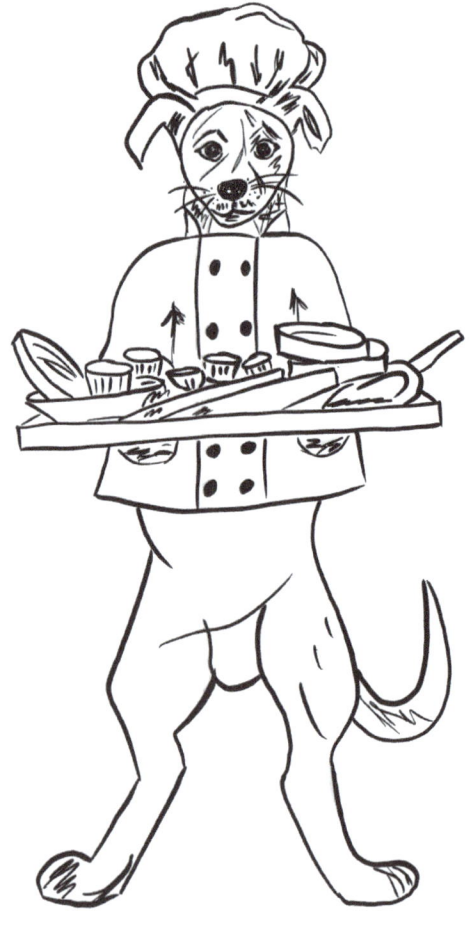

BAKING DISH EQUIVALENTS

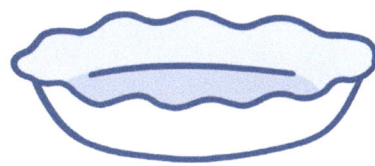

9 by 1 ½-inch pie pan = 5 cups
9 ½ by 2-inch deep-dish pie pan = 7 cups

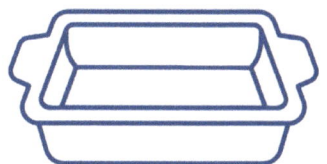

8 by 8 by 2-inch square pan = 8 cups
9 by 9 by 1 ½-inch square pan = 8 cups
9 by 9 by 2-inch square pan= 10 cups

8 ½ by 4 ½ by 2 ½ -inch loaf pan = 6 cups
9 by 5 by 3-inch loaf pan = 8 cups

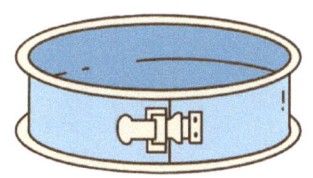

9-inch by 2-inch depth cake pan = 8 cups
9 ½ by 2 ½-inch springform pans = 10 cups

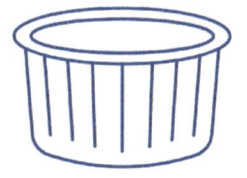

Common ramekins are about 4-inches in diameter by 2-inches in depth. which = about ¾ cup and 1 cup respectively

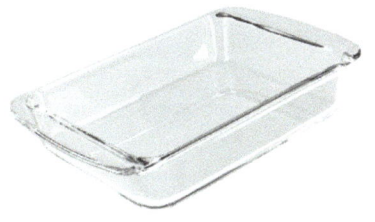

8 ½ by 11 by 2-inch baking dish = 8 cups
9 by 13 by 2-inch baking dish = 12 cups
12 ¼ by 8 ¾ by 2 ½-inch oval dish = 8 cups

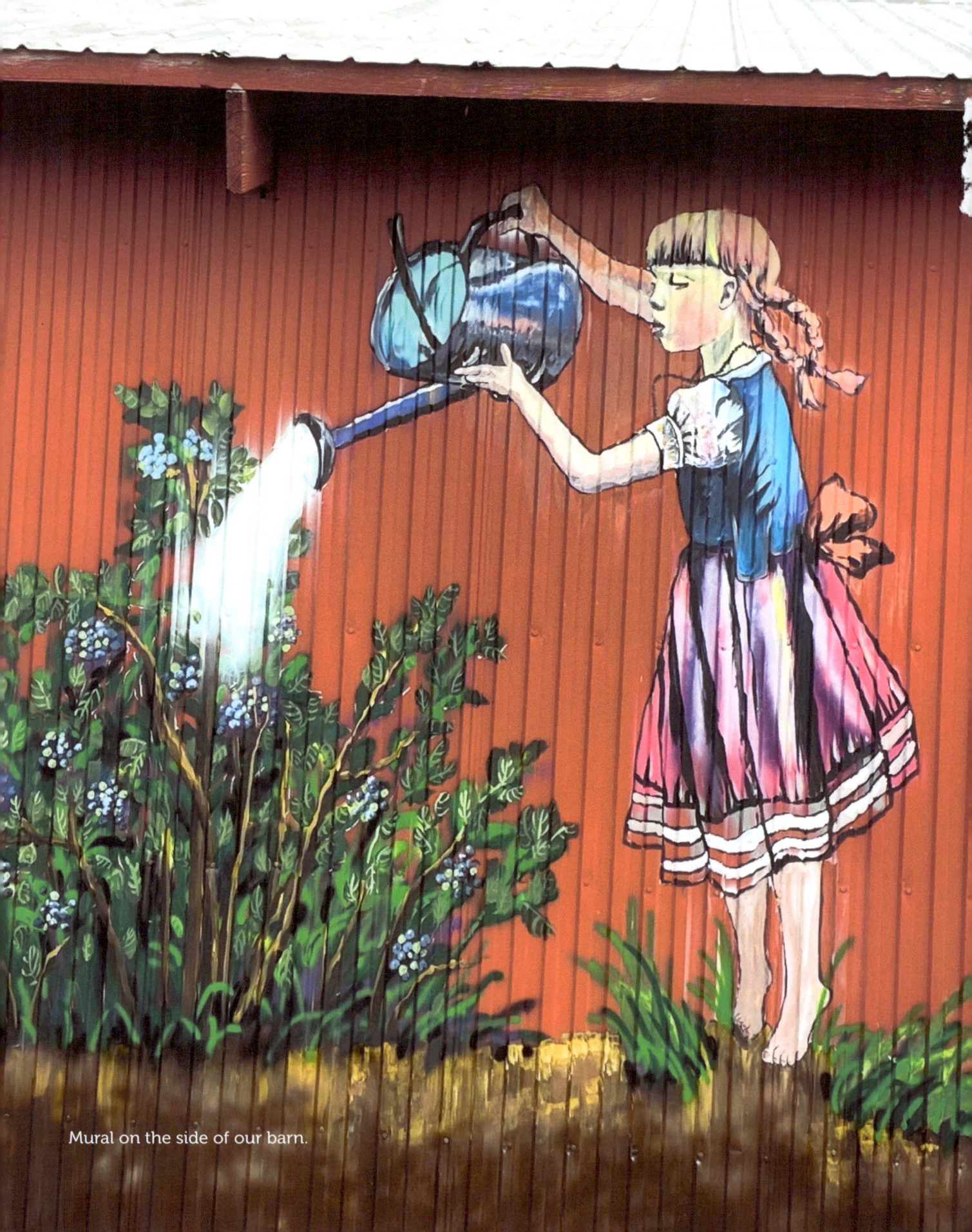
Mural on the side of our barn.

Blueberries 101

WHEN TO USE FROZEN VS FRESH

Most of the baking recipes in this cookbook were made with slightly thawed frozen blueberries. This was partially to prevent them from bleeding into the baked goods, and partially because I was developing the recipes in the early spring before fresh blueberries were ready to harvest in Minnesota.

What I found when working with blueberries is that the baking recipes actually turned out better using frozen berries—no bleeding and sweeter berries due to being frozen in their prime.

When fresh or dried blueberries were required for the recipe (such as chicken dinner salad or blueberry scones), I will note that in the ingredient list.

TO THAW OR NOT TO THAW...

Most of the baked goods recipes in this book used partially thawed frozen blueberries. By partially thawed, I mean I took them out of the freezer and let them sit on the counter for a few minutes, just long enough to get any ice off. Alternatively, you can quickly rinse the frozen berries with cold water to remove the ice and then pat them dry.

Do not thaw blueberries for recipes that have long cook times. This will help prevent both color bleeding and a soggy texture.

Some cookbooks recommend tossing frozen berries with a tablespoon of flour before adding them to the batter. This is to prevent them from sinking to the bottom. I did not find this to be a necessary step. Each recipe has a finished photo that shows you what the end result looks like, and none of them "sank" to the bottom.

When incorporating blueberries into a batter, make sure to stir them in gently. This is what is meant by 'folding'. The goal is to avoid breaking their skin, which will release too much juice.

Note: frozen blueberries can lower the temperature of the batter, so you may need to increase the baking time by a few minutes. Always test by inserting a toothpick or metal tester into the batter, as cooking times vary with each individual oven.

WHAT TO LOOK FOR WHEN PURCHASING FRESH BLUEBERRIES

If you want to avoid tart blueberries, avoid the reddish/purple color on the blossom end. Those are berries that were harvested before becoming completely ripe and they will be much tarter. Blueberries do not ripen after harvesting.

The silvery, dusty color on fresh blueberries is a natural coating that actually indicates freshness. It does not indicate spoilage.

Check the container for juice stains, as that may mean the berries were not handled carefully and might be damaged. Also check for mold, of course, and discard those that show signs of mold.

ADDING SUGAR TO BLUEBERRY RECIPES

There are several situations where adding sugar can benefit the flavor or texture of recipes using blueberries. Here are the most important:

Macerating for syrups and jellies

Adding sugar to blueberries and allowing them to sit for a while (macerating), will draw out their juices and create softened, juicy berries. Draining these softened berries through a fine-mesh sieve will give you a sweet syrup that can be used in syrups or jellies.

Cooking on the stovetop

Adding sugar to berries in a saucepan and gently cooking with other ingredients like lemon juice or spices is needed to create a compote, sauce or jam.

Baked goods will require some amount of sugar for flavor and structure. Decreasing the sugar too much from pies, muffins, and cakes can result in an unsuccessful dish.

FREEZING AND STORING

Freezing

First spread them in a single layer on a cookie sheet (also called a sheet pan). Freeze them solid, which may take several hours. Then transfer them to freezer bags for long-term storage. Label and date the bags, and remove as much air as possible before placing them in the freezer.

Do not rinse before freezing. Blueberries have a natural protective coating that you don't want to wash away.

Blueberries can keep for a year or more if properly frozen. If you notice freezer burn on your berries, they are still usable but the flavor might be diminished.

Storing fresh berries

Before storing them in your refrigerator, sort the berries and remove any that are mushy or moldy. Do not wash them until ready to use.

Store them in a breathable container, and do not place them in the crisper drawer, as it is too humid.

Fresh berries should last 3-5 days in the refrigerator if they were harvested properly. If they start to get soft or mushy, consider freezing them.

GOOD FLAVOR PAIRINGS

Blueberries pair well with a wide range of spices and other fruits. Some of my favorites are listed below. For an in-depth look at blueberry pairings check out "The Flavor Bible" by Karen Page and Andrew Dornenburg.

Citrus Pairings

Lemon and lime for added tartness and orange for sweetness.

Fruit Pairings

Blackberries for a beautiful color combination, and strawberries and raspberries for enhanced berry flavor.

Spice and Herb Pairings

Cinnamon and cardamom for warmth; basil or mint for fresh summer flavors; lavender or vanilla for sweetness or aromatic enhancement.

Other great pairings

Balsamic vinegar is great for balancing the sweetness of blueberries; mascarpone and many dairy products are great pairings for a creamy base.

GROWING YOUR OWN BLUEBERRIES

Learning to grow your own blueberries, whether in a garden or a pot, is a book unto itself. I have over 20 years of experience growing blueberries in the Midwest, and I hope to share that experience in an upcoming book.

For now, however, I would refer you to the Resource Page at the back of this cookbook, where you will find links to a wide range of articles that are specific to growing blueberries.

There is nothing like cooking with homegrown fruit or vegetables. In addition to the optimal flavor you can achieve, the self-confidence of growing your own food can't be beat. There is definitely a learning curve with growing blueberries, but I would encourage you to explore the possibilities.

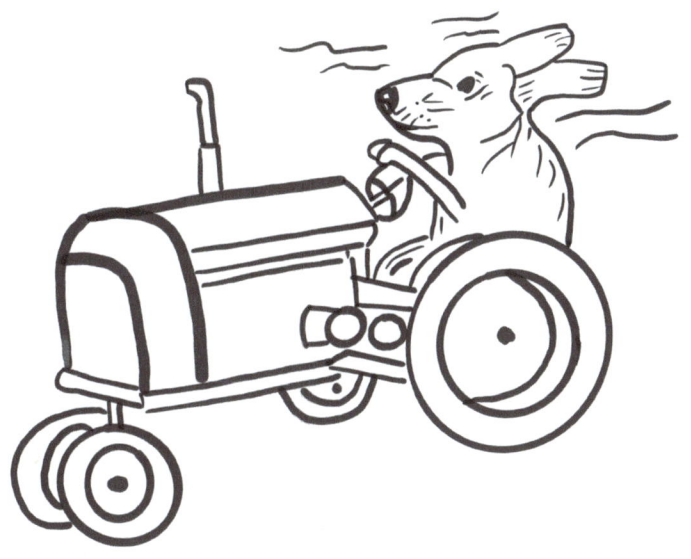

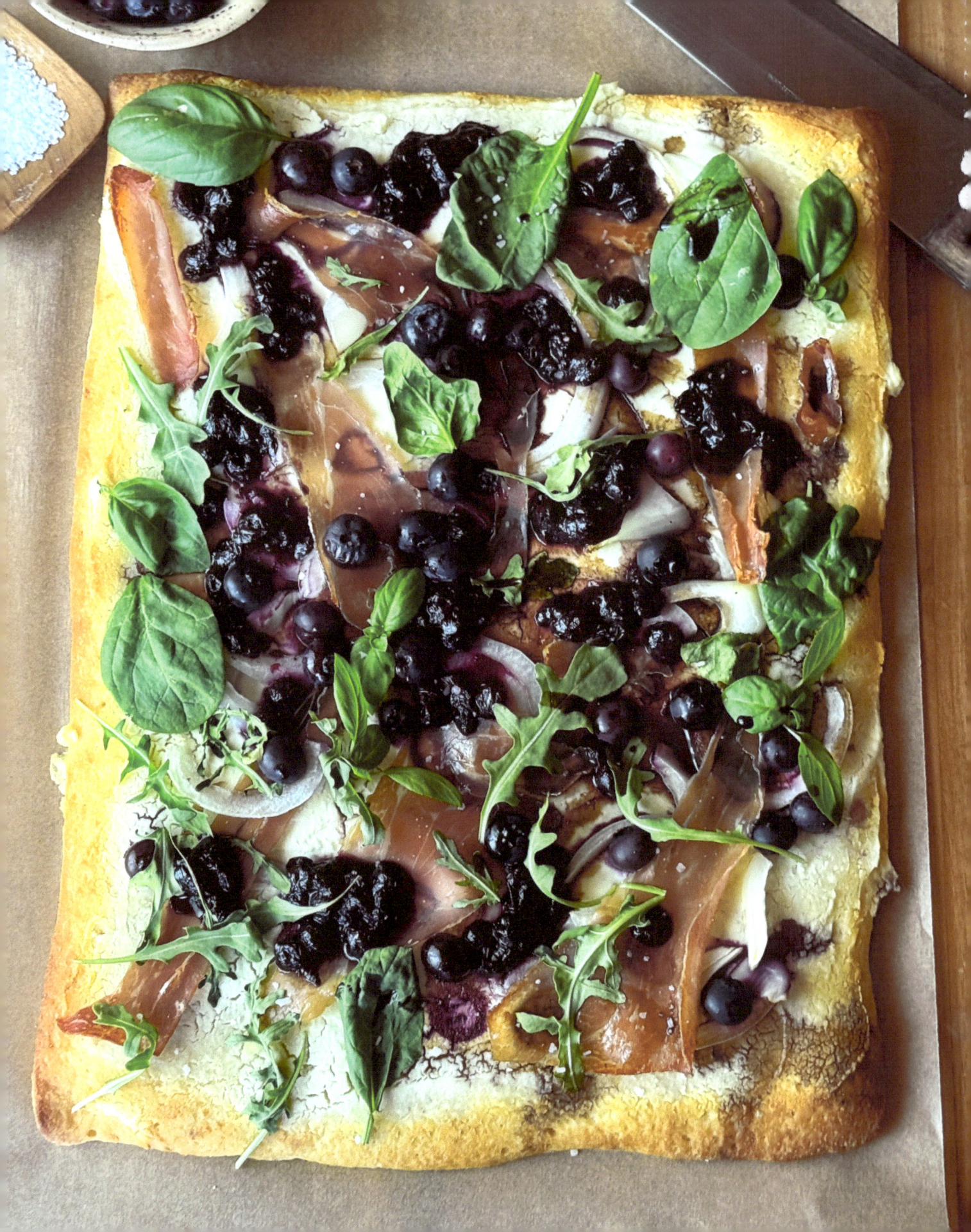

Part II
Let's Cook

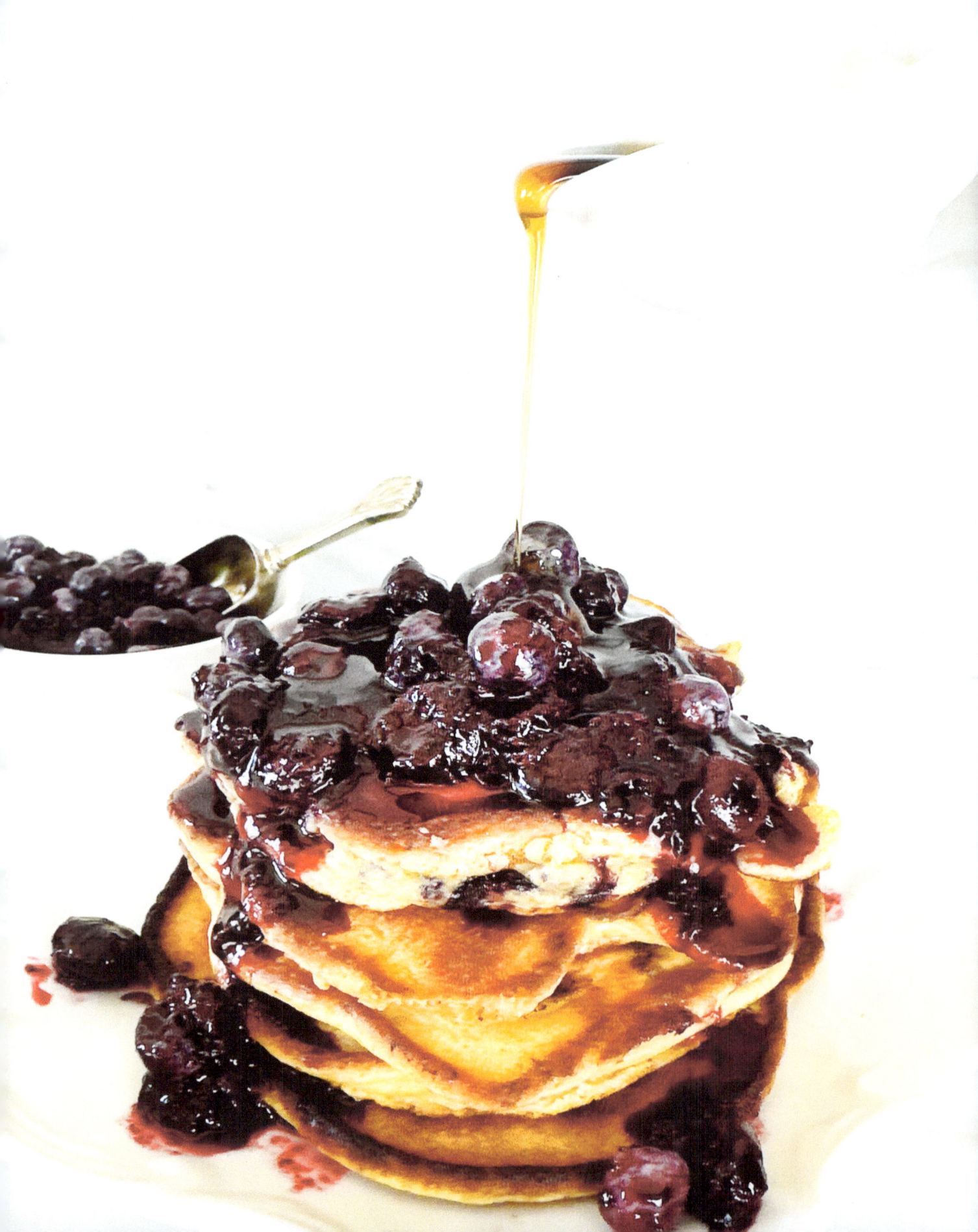

BREAKFAST

- High-Protein Blueberry Mint Smoothie
- Overnight Steel Cut Oatmeal
- 4 Easy Blueberry Toast Variations
- Breakfast Popsicles
- Blueberry Zucchini Bread
- Fluffy Pancakes with Blueberry Topping
- Dutch Baby: Oven Baked
- Make Ahead French Toast Casserole
- Blueberry Ginger Lime Muffins
- Bakery Style Blueberry Muffins with Cinnamon Crumb Topping
- Blueberry Scones with Earl Grey Tea & Lavender
- Breakfast Crepes with Ricotta Filling & Blueberry Topping

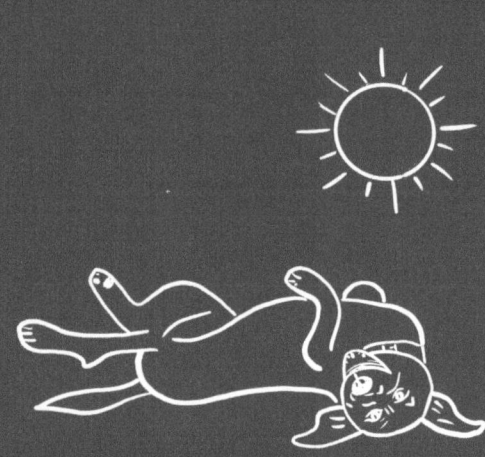

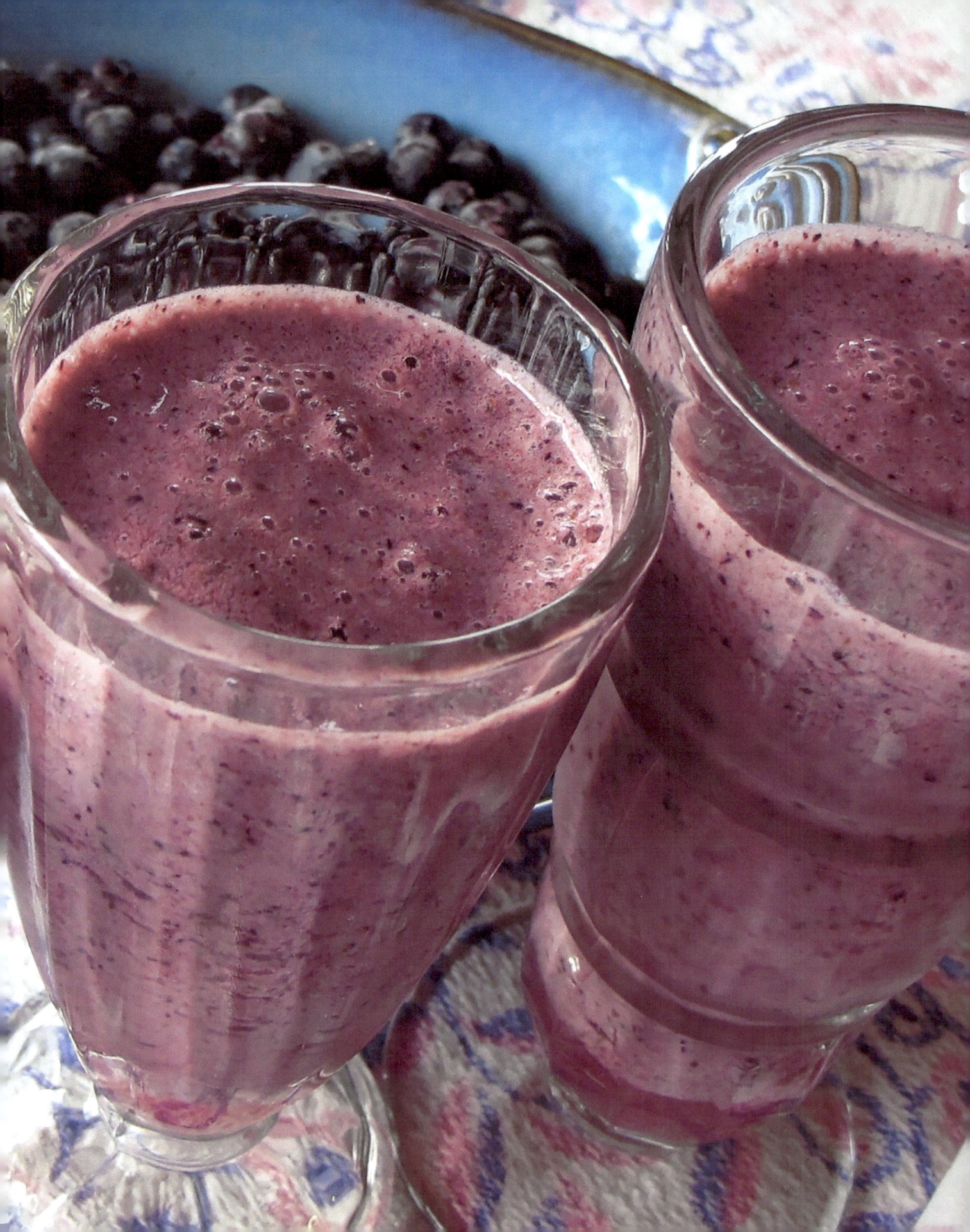

EASY — Makes one 10-oz glass

High-Protein Blueberry Mint Smoothie

I followed a slow carb diet for many years and this high protein smoothie was my daily go-to breakfast. It kept me full and energetic for most of the day, and I never felt deprived on the flavor front! Blueberries and mint are the winning combination here, but feel free to leave out the protein powder if you're not a fan.

INGREDIENTS

½ cup (120ml) unsweetened coconut milk

1 cup water (240ml)

½ cup ice cubes

½ cup (3oz) frozen blueberries

1 oz (28g) whey protein powder

1 tablespoon chia seeds

2-3 sprigs of fresh mint (about 10-12 leaves)

1 cup fresh spinach leaves (packed)

SUBSTITUTIONS & ADDITIONS

- Substitute almond milk for coconut milk.
- Substitute any of your favorite greens for spinach.
- Strawberries are a good substitute for blueberries; blackberries and raspberries tend to be seedy.
- Avocados can be added for the fat if you don't want milk.
- 1-2 tablespoons peanut butter is a good addition for more protein.
- Cottage cheese can stand in for milk.
- Cacao nibs can add richness.

DIRECTIONS

1. Add milk and water to a blender, then add ice cubes, blueberries, protein powder, chia seeds, mint and spinach (don't worry, you won't taste the spinach). Blend all ingredients until smooth.
2. Pour into a large glass and enjoy.
3. Rinse your blender with hot water right away, as the mixture is hard to clean once dried.

COOKING NOTES

Low-carb notes:

- Berries and avocados are the main fruits that work for strict low-carb diets. Avoid high-sugar bananas. You can get a thick texture from frozen blueberries and ice cubes.
- Don't substitute water for milk if you are practicing a low carb diet, as the fat in the milk is what keeps you satiated until your next meal.
- If you opt out of protein powder, you might want to add a little sweetener, as protein powder often contains sweeteners that help balance the tartness of the berries.

Nutrition Notes: Calories 226; Protein 31g; Carbs 15g; Fat 5g; Sugar 13g

MODERATE — Makes 3-4 servings; Overnight refrigeration required

Overnight Steel Cut Oatmeal

I grew up with cereal for breakfast—usually cold sugary cereal, but sometimes warm Malt-O-Meal and occasionally oatmeal. When I had kids of my own, I thought steel cut oatmeal would be the healthy breakfast answer, but it felt like such a production in the morning. Instant oats were quick, but they were basically fast food masquerading as health food. Nobody wanted that mushy mess.

Fast forward to visiting my adult son in Denver, who is a bona fide health enthusiast. We stopped at an upscale restaurant for breakfast and I ordered oatmeal on a whim. To my surprise, it was a nutty, creamy, satisfying bowl of oatmeal. It became a food memory that I had to recreate as soon as I got home. The bonus of overnight oatmeal is that it is actually doable on busy mornings.

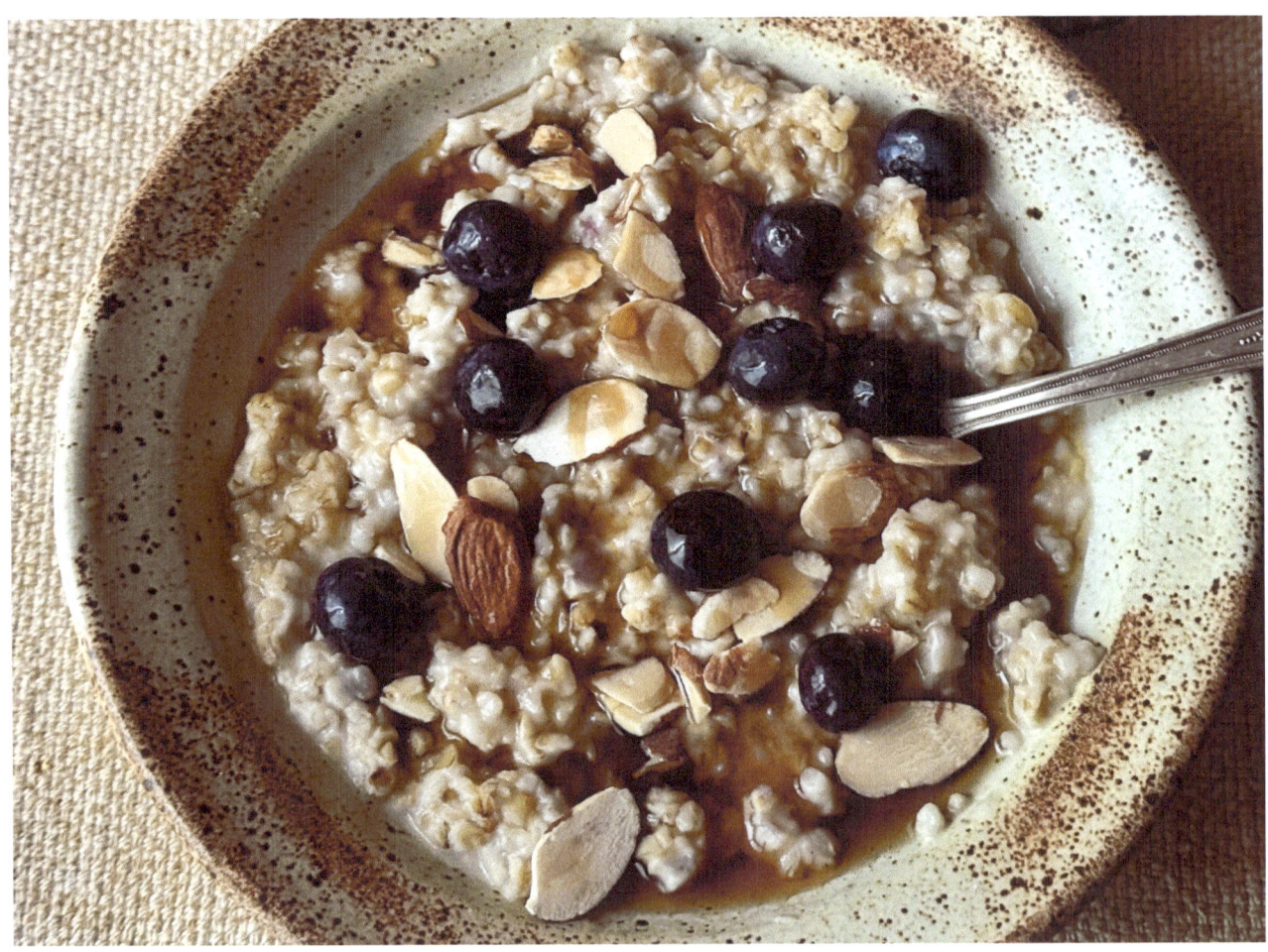

INGREDIENTS

1 teaspoon unsalted butter

1 cup (5 oz) steel cut oats

3 cups (710 ml) water

¼ teaspoon kosher salt

1 teaspoon cinnamon

1 teaspoon vanilla

½ cup (120 ml) milk

1 tablespoon brown sugar

½ cup (3 oz) blueberries

SUBSTITUTIONS & ADDITIONS

- Don't substitute rolled oats for steel cut oats in this recipe—they have completely different textures and cooking times. Steel cut oats stay chewy and never get mushy, which is exactly what makes this recipe special.
- Substitute honey, maple syrup or agave nectar for the brown sugar.
- Substitute your favorite non-dairy milk.

ABOUT STEEL CUT OATS

- Steel cut oats are also known as Irish oats or pinhead oats.
- They are made by cutting oat groats into pieces, rather than rolling or flattening them.
- Steel cut oats are higher in fiber than regular rolled oats. They tend to keep you satiated for a longer period of time.

DIRECTIONS

1. Melt the butter over medium heat in a saucepan that is large enough to accommodate 4 cups of oatmeal with spare room at the top (about 3 quarts). Add the oats to the hot butter and toast them for about 3 minutes, or until you start to smell a nutty aroma.

2. Add the water, salt, cinnamon and vanilla. Bring to a boil, and continue boiling for 1 minute, then remove from heat. Stir, cover the pan, and let it sit overnight at room temperature.

3. The next morning, uncover and bring to a gentle simmer (small bubbles) over medium heat. Stir in the milk and heat through, adding more milk if you prefer a creamier texture.

4. Serve in bowls topped with brown sugar and blueberries.

5. Refrigerate any leftovers, covered, for up to 5 days. Their texture will soften more each day. Just reheat a bowl at a time, adding more milk if desired and your preferred amount of sugar and blueberries.

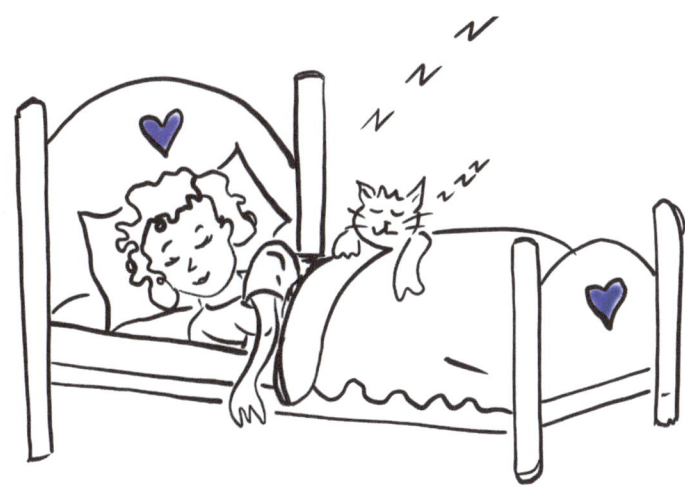

Nutrition Notes: Calories 204; Protein 8g; Carbs 32g; Fat 4g; Sugar 4g

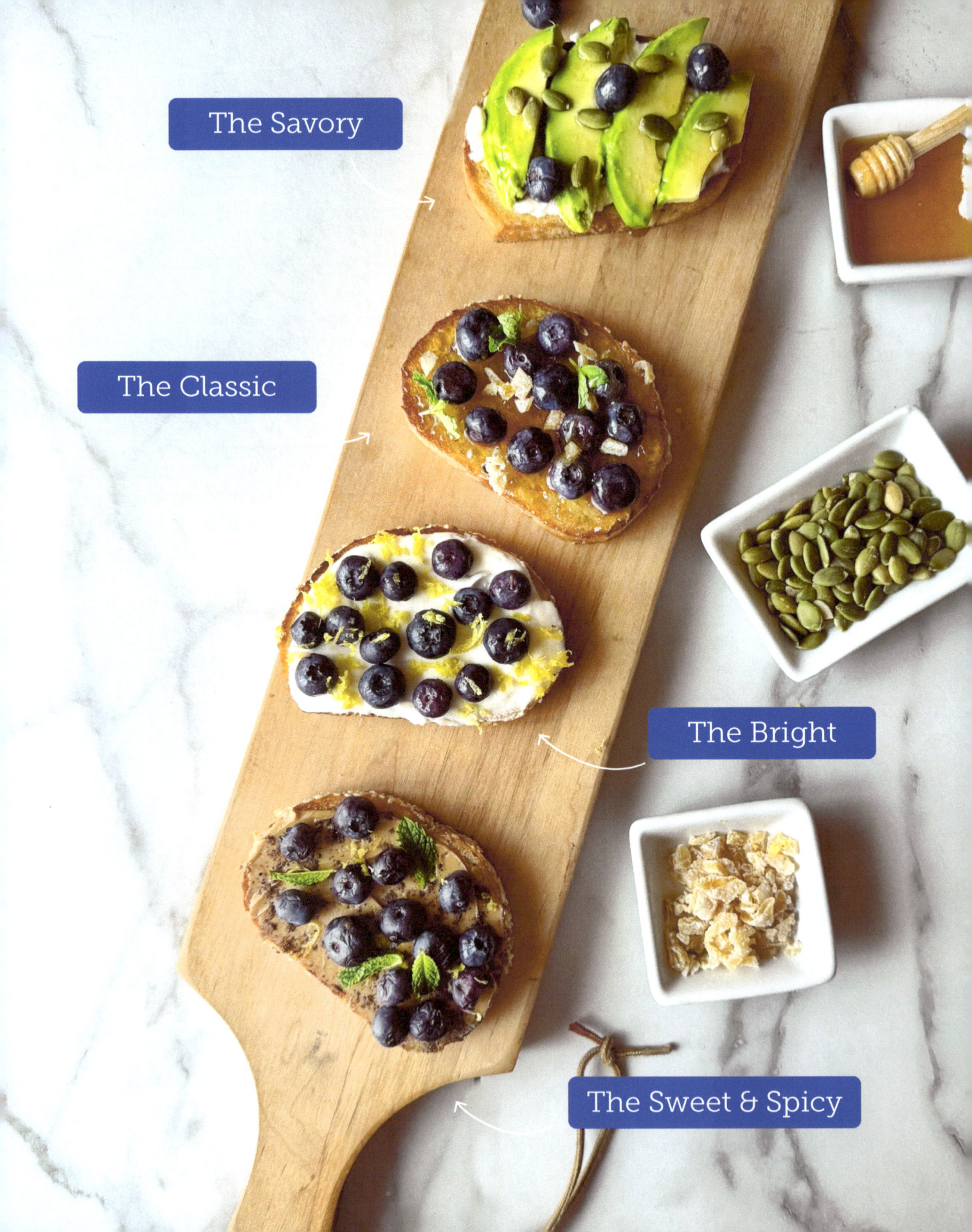

🥄 EASY — 1 serving = 1 slice of toast

4 Easy Bluberry Toast Variations

In a rush to get out the door in the morning, but want something more substantial (and healthy) than the stale muffin from the grocery store? Try one of these quick and easy options. You won't be disappointed in the flavor and you'll stay satiated until lunchtime! Happiness all-around.

• •

TEMPLATE FOR BLUEBERRY TOAST

Here's the basic formula for building the perfect blueberry toast:

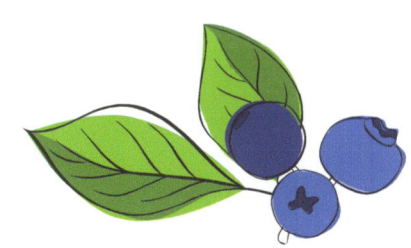

Choose Your Base (something sturdy):
  Rye, sourdough, 7-grain or multigrain
  Avoid soft white breads like brioche

Add a Creamy Layer:
  Nut butters (peanut, almond)
  Avocado
  Cottage cheese or Greek yogurt
  Ricotta, goat cheese or cream cheese
  Jam

Top with Blueberries:
  Fresh or frozen

  If the berries are tart, drizzle with honey, maple syrup, or a sprinkle of cinnamon

Finish with a Flair:
  Citrus zest (lemon or lime)
  Dried blueberries or craisins
  Pepitas (pumpkin seeds)
  Minced candied ginger
  Mint, sage or your favorite herb
  Chile crisp (or spicy chili powder)

MY FOUR FAVORITES

1. **The Savory:** Cottage cheese + mashed avocado + blueberries + pepitas

2. **The Sweet & Spicy:** Peanut butter + honey + blueberries + minced candied ginger

3. **The Bright:** Lemon yogurt + blueberries + fresh lemon zest

4. **The Classic:** Orange marmalade + blueberries + fresh mint

COOKING NOTES

Can't find lemon yogurt? Just stir fresh lemon juice into plain Greek yogurt—start with a teaspoon and adjust to taste.

Nutrition Notes: Values vary by combination. Range per serving: Calories 185-310; Protein 4-16g; Values for Avocado Toast Variation: Calories 328; Protein 11g; Carbs 26g; Fat 11g; Sugar 7g

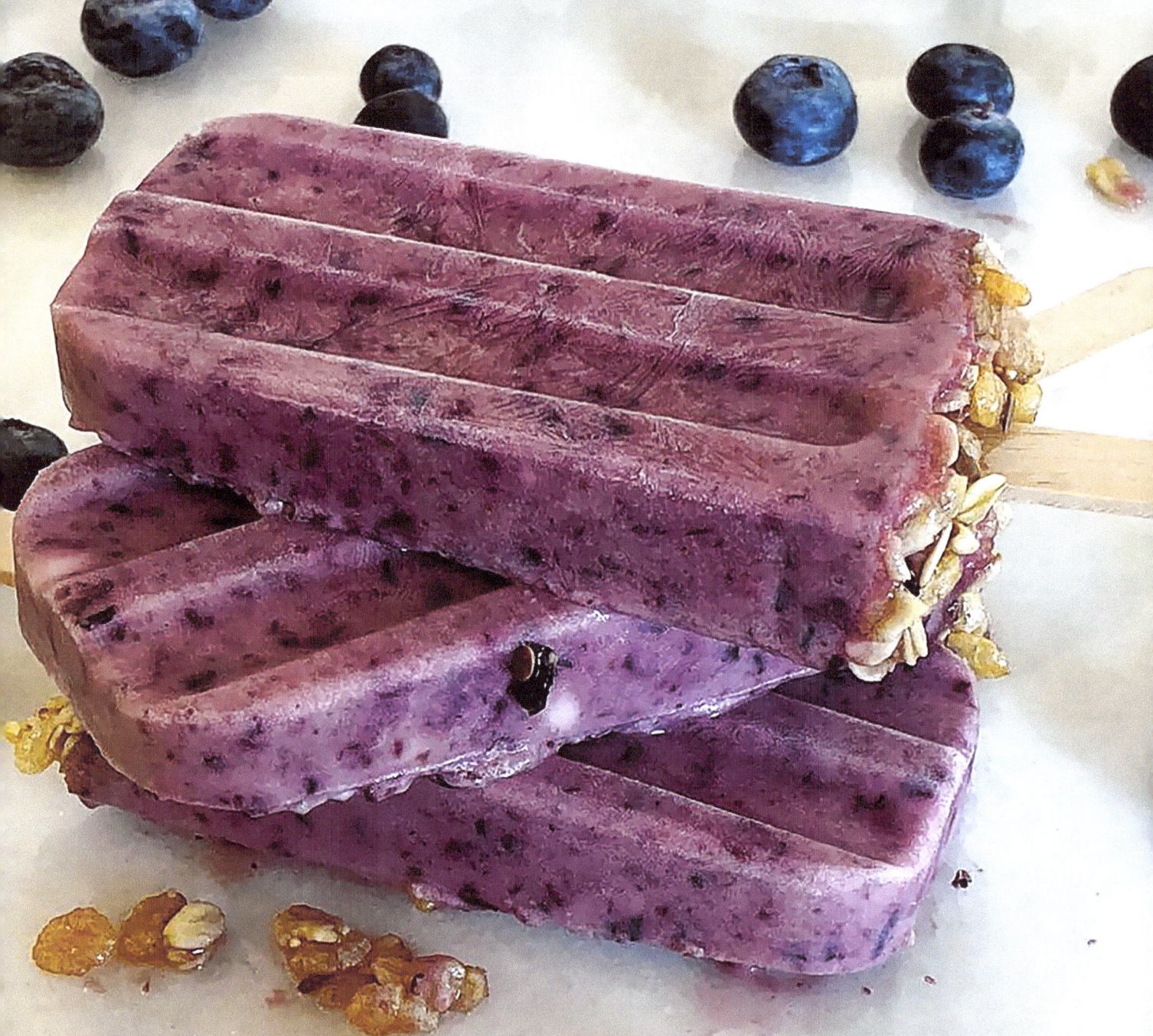

COOKING NOTES

- Full-fat yogurt will give you a creamier texture and low-fat yogurt will result in an icier texture.
- Popsicles will keep in the freezer for up to 2 months.
- If you don't have popsicle molds, use small paper cups and wooden sticks—just cover with foil and poke the sticks through.

🥄 EASY — Makes 4 popsicles; Needs freezing time of 4+ hours

Blueberry Yogurt Breakfast Popsicles

Who says you can't have popsicles for breakfast? These aren't your typical sugar-bomb frozen treats—they're packed with protein-rich Greek yogurt, antioxidant-loaded blueberries, crunchy granola, and just enough sweetness to make mornings feel like a celebration. Make these ahead and you'll have a perfectly nutritious breakfast before hitting the beach. Bonus—kids love them!

• •

INGREDIENTS

1 ½ cups (9oz) blueberries (thawed if using frozen)

2 tablespoons jam or jelly

1 ½ cups (360g) greek plain yogurt

3-4 tablespoons granola

1 tablespoon honey

SUBSTITUTIONS & ADDITIONS

- Substitute chopped nuts for granola.
- Substitute different berries for the blueberries.
- Substitute full-fat coconut milk for yogurt.
- Add 2 tablespoons lime juice for a punch of freshness.
- Add 1 teaspoon vanilla for more sweetness.
- Add 1 tablespoon chia seeds to the granola base for extra fiber.

DIRECTIONS

1. In a food processor or blender purée the blueberries and the jam until smooth and creamy.

2. Vigorously whisk the yogurt in a bowl to remove any clumps.

3. Gently combine the blueberry purée and the yogurt in a large bowl, making swirls if you like. Don't overmix or you'll lose the swirl effect.

4. Fill the popsicle molds ¾ full with the yogurt mixture, leaving room for expansion during freezing. Then sprinkle granola on top and drizzle with honey to help it adhere. Insert popsicle sticks.

5. Place in the freezer for at least 4 hours. When ready to eat one, run warm water over the outside of the mold for 10-20 seconds and gently wiggle the stick back and forth until popsicle is released. Enjoy!

Nutrition Notes (per 1 popsicle): Calories 55; Protein 4g; Carbs 9g; Fat 1g; Sugar 6g

EASY — Makes one 9- by 5-inch loaf (about 14 slices)

Blueberry Zucchini Bread with Lemon Icing

An overabundance of zucchini and an easy one-bowl recipe make this quick bread a summertime favorite for a grab-and-go breakfast. I tested this recipe 3 times trying to figure out what the slightly bitter aftertaste was. Turns out it was the baking soda. I backed off the amount of baking soda and the final loaf was everything zucchini bread should be—easy, delicious, portable, and on the healthier side with the added blueberries.

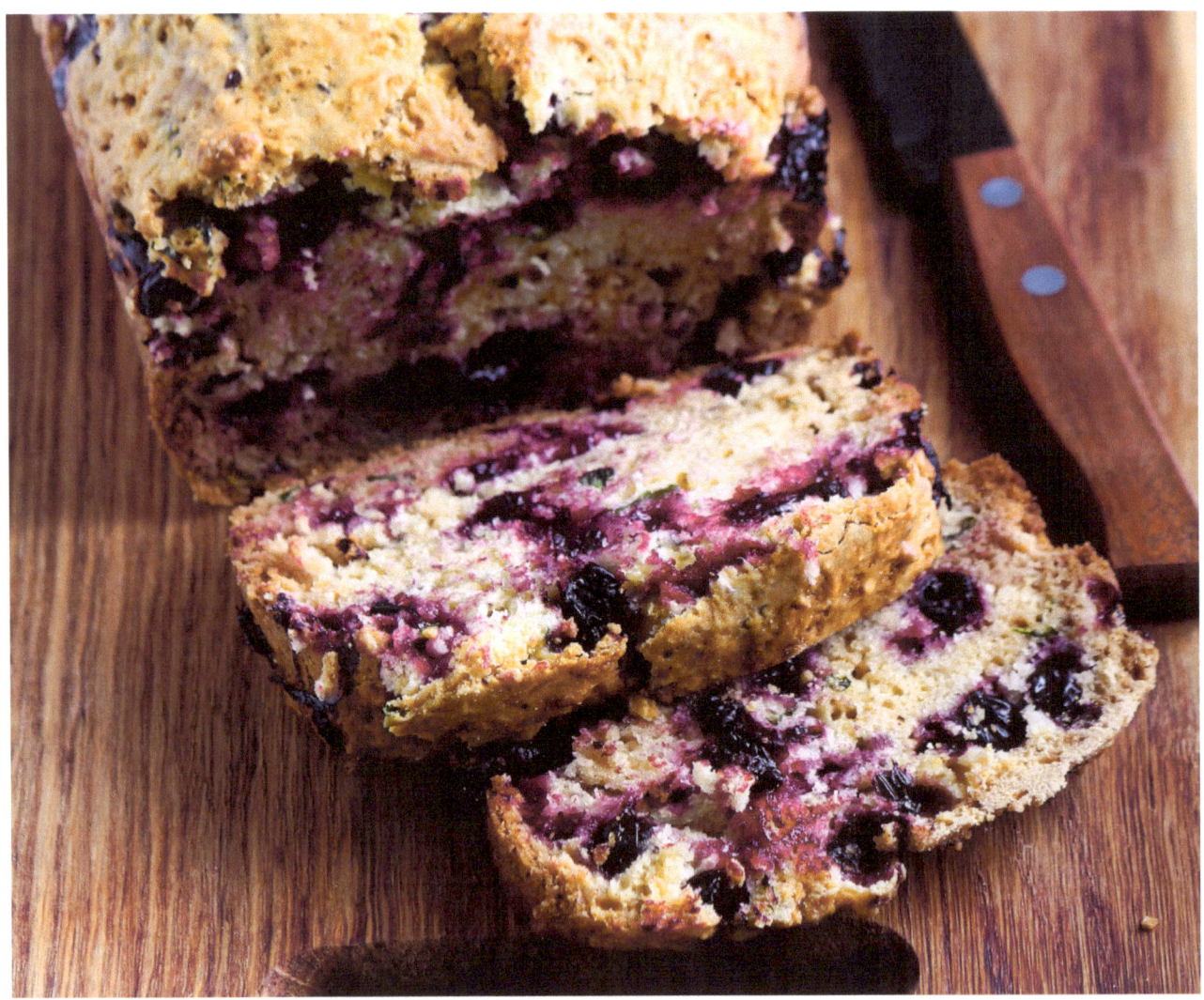

INGREDIENTS

For the bread:

1 ½ cups (150 g) shredded zucchini (one small zucchini)

½ cup (100 g) granulated sugar

¼ cup (55 g) brown sugar, packed

½ cup (119 ml) vegetable oil

2 eggs

1 teaspoon vanilla

2 teaspoons lemon zest

2 teaspoons lemon juice

1 ½ cups (185 g) all-purpose flour

½ teaspoon baking soda

½ teaspoon baking powder

½ teaspoon kosher salt

1 teaspoon cinnamon

1 cup (6 oz) blueberries (fresh or frozen)

For the glaze:

1 cup powdered sugar

4 teaspoons fresh lemon juice

2 teaspoons lemon zest for garnish (optional)

SUBSTITUTIONS & ADDITIONS

1. Add ½ cup of nuts to the batter for a crunch.
2. Substitute ½ cup brown sugar and ¼ cup white granulated sugar for the ¾ cup granulated sugar.
3. Add ⅓ cup mini chocolate chips for added sweetness.

DIRECTIONS

1. Preheat the oven to 350°F (176°C). Grease a 9- by 5-inch loaf pan with cooking spray or butter.
2. Rinse and dry a small zucchini. Use the large holes in a box grater to shred the zucchini and measure out 1 ½ cups. Set aside.
3. In a large bowl, whisk together both sugars, oil, eggs, vanilla, lemon zest, and lemon juice.
4. In another bowl, whisk together the dry ingredients (flour, baking soda, baking powder, salt and cinnamon).
5. Stir the flour mixture into the bowl of wet ingredients and mix until thoroughly combined. Add the zucchini to the bowl and mix until evenly distributed. Gently fold in the blueberries, being careful not to break the skins so they don't bleed.
6. Using a spatula, add the batter to the prepared loaf pan.
7. Bake for 55-65 minutes, or until a knife inserted into the middle of the loaf comes out clean.
8. Transfer the loaf bread to a wire rack to cool. While the bread is cooling, make the glaze by stirring together the powdered sugar and the lemon juice.
9. When the loaf bread has cooled for 10-15 minutes, remove it from the pan and drizzle the glaze over the top, letting it run down the sides. Sprinkle with garnish of lemon zest (optional).

Nutrition Notes (per slice): Calories 178; Protein 3g; Carbs 23g; Fat 9g; Sugar 12g

MODERATE — Makes 12-13 pancakes using ¼ cup batter per pancake; Topping makes 2 cups

Fluffy Pancakes with Blueberry Topping

These pancakes are what happens when Italian comfort food meets American breakfast tradition. The ricotta creates fluffy, cloud-like pancakes that are almost custard-y in the center, while the blueberry compote bursts with bright, jammy sweetness. Sure, they take a bit more effort than mixing batter up from a box, but one bite and you'll understand why breakfast enthusiasts love this recipe. Perfect for a lazy Sunday morning or for showing houseguests they are special to you.

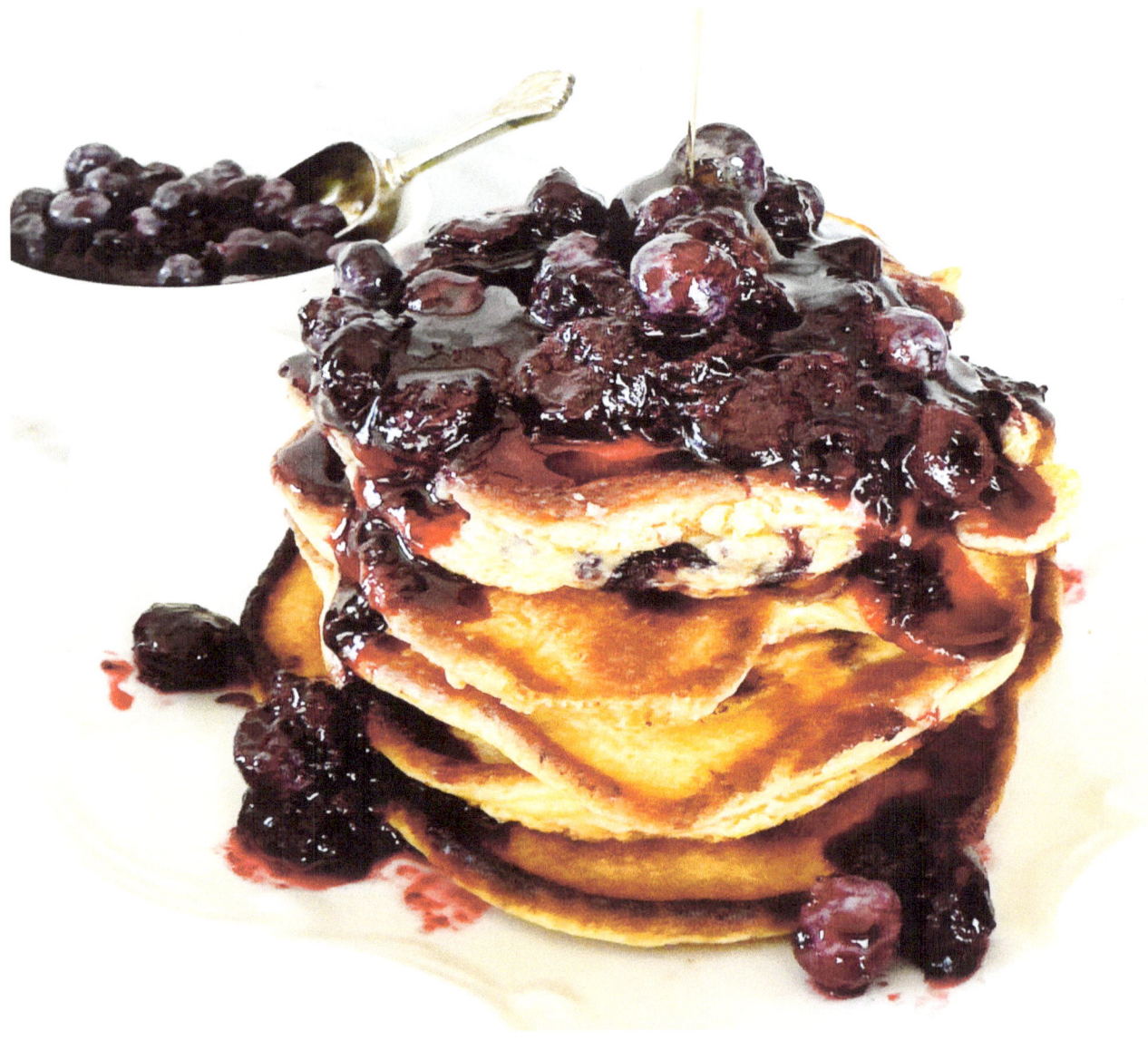

INGREDIENTS

For the Pancakes:

- ¾ cups (225g) ricotta cheese (full fat)
- 3 large eggs
- 3 tablespoons granulated sugar
- ¾ cup (180ml) milk
- ½ teaspoon vanilla extract
- 1 teaspoon white vinegar
- 1⅓ (187g) cups all-purpose flour
- 2 teaspoons baking powder
- ¼ teaspoon baking soda
- ¼ teaspoon kosher salt
- 1-2 teaspoons unsalted butter

For the Topping:

- 3 cups (18oz) blueberries
- ¼ cup (50g) sugar
- ⅛ teaspoon salt
- 1 ½ teaspoon lemon zest
- 1 tablespoon fresh lemon juice

SUBSTITUTIONS & ADDITIONS

- Do not substitute whipped or creamed ricotta for full fat ricotta
- Substitute orange zest & juice for the lemon in the compote
- These pancakes won't dry out due to the ricotta, but they need to cook long enough to ensure they are cooked inside. 3-5 minutes is the sweet spot.
- Don't overdo the butter between batches or the cakes will come out with uneven browning (or burnt butter)
- Pancakes will keep 3 months in the freezer.

DIRECTIONS

Make the Blueberry Topping:

1. To a medium saucepan, add 2 cups blueberries, ¼ cup sugar and ⅛ teaspoon salt. Cook over medium heat until berries burst and the mixture thickens (about 6-8 minutes).
2. Add lemon zest, lemon juice and remaining blueberries to the pan and bring to a boil. Remove from heat right after it boils. Set aside.

Make the Pancakes:

3. In a large bowl, vigorously whisk the first 6 ingredients together (cheese, eggs, sugar, milk, vanilla, and vinegar). Small curds of the ricotta are okay.
4. Whisk the dry ingredients (flour, baking powder, baking soda and salt) together in a separate bowl. Fold the dry ingredients into the larger bowl of wet ingredients. The batter will be slightly thick due to the ricotta.
5. Melt a little butter in a skillet over medium heat and then pour in ¼ cup of the batter and let it spread, gently spreading it into a circle with the back of a spoon.
6. Cook the first side for 1-2 minutes or until bottoms are golden brown and a few bubbles form on top. Flip and cook about 2 minutes longer, reducing heat if they are browning too quickly.
7. Transfer to a heat proof plate and place in a 200°F (90°C) oven to keep warm.
8. Repeat the process adding a little butter in between cooking each batch.
9. Serve with warm blueberry compote, maple syrup and room temperature butter.

Nutrition Notes (for 1 pancake-topping included): Calories 148; Protein 6g; Carbs 18g; Fat 6g; Sugar 5g

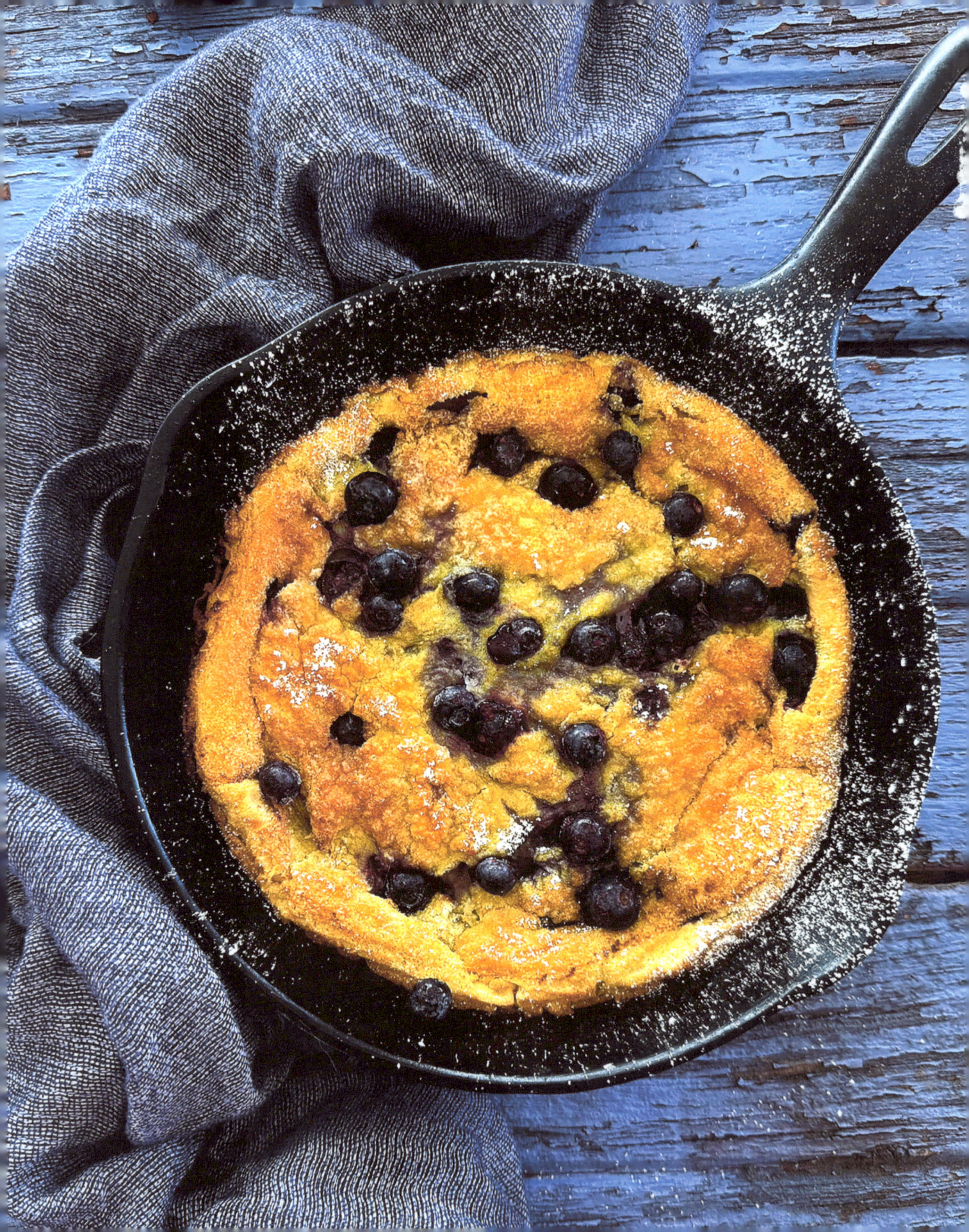

EASY — (if you have a blender) — Makes one 10-inch diameter pancake (6 wedges)

Dutch Baby: Oven Baked

Imagine a giant, blueberry-studded pancake with a puffy golden brown crust and a creamy, custardy center. That's a Dutch baby— the show-stopping breakfast that makes you look like a culinary genius with surprisingly little effort.

INGREDIENTS

⅔ cup (160ml) milk, room temp.

4 large eggs, room temp.

½ cup (73g) all purpose flour

1 tablespoon orange zest (or lemon zest)

1 teaspoon vanilla

¼ teaspoon kosher salt

4 tablespoons unsalted butter

1 cup (6oz) blueberries, frozen are fine

2 tablespoons powdered sugar

COOKING NOTES

- For a 12-inch skillet, increase all ingredients by 25%.
- Check frequently so it doesn't burn, as all oven temperatures are different.
- Let ingredients come to room temperature before starting for best results.
- Frozen berries will not bleed as much if used straight from the freezer.
- Cast iron skillets work best as they provide even heating.

DIRECTIONS

1. **Preheat the oven to 425°F (220°C).** Place empty 9-10 inch skillet in oven to heat up while oven is preheating.
2. Add milk, eggs, flour, zest, vanilla, and salt to a blender and blend on high speed for one minute, or until thoroughly smooth.
3. Remove the skillet from the oven and add the butter to the skillet. It will bubble and turn a light brown and that is fine. Spread the butter up the sides of the skillet using a spatula or pastry brush.
4. Pour the batter from the blender into the center of the skillet. Sprinkle the blueberries evenly over the batter.
5. Transfer the skillet to the preheated oven and bake about 20 minutes, or until golden brown. Don't open the oven during the first 15 minutes so that the Dutch baby will puff up, but do check after 15 minutes to prevent burning, as oven temperatures vary. It takes about 20 minutes in a 9- to 10-inch skillet.
6. When edges are golden brown, carefully remove from the oven. It will deflate slightly as it cools.
7. Sift some powdered sugar over the Dutch baby and enjoy with a side of maple syrup or blueberry jam.

Nutrition Notes (per serving): Calories 188; Protein 6g; Carbs 16g; Fat 11g; Sugar 7g

MODERATE — Makes one 9 x 13-inch casserole (8 large servings)

Make Ahead French Toast Casserole

Who doesn't want to make their life easier with a make-ahead breakfast? Especially one that looks elegant, tastes delightful, and is super easy (both the prep and the baking). These popular make-ahead casseroles are becoming classics for Christmas morning, but why wait for a holiday? Make any morning a mellow time for the cook with a delicious French toast recipe that doesn't require standing over the stove tending to individual slices.

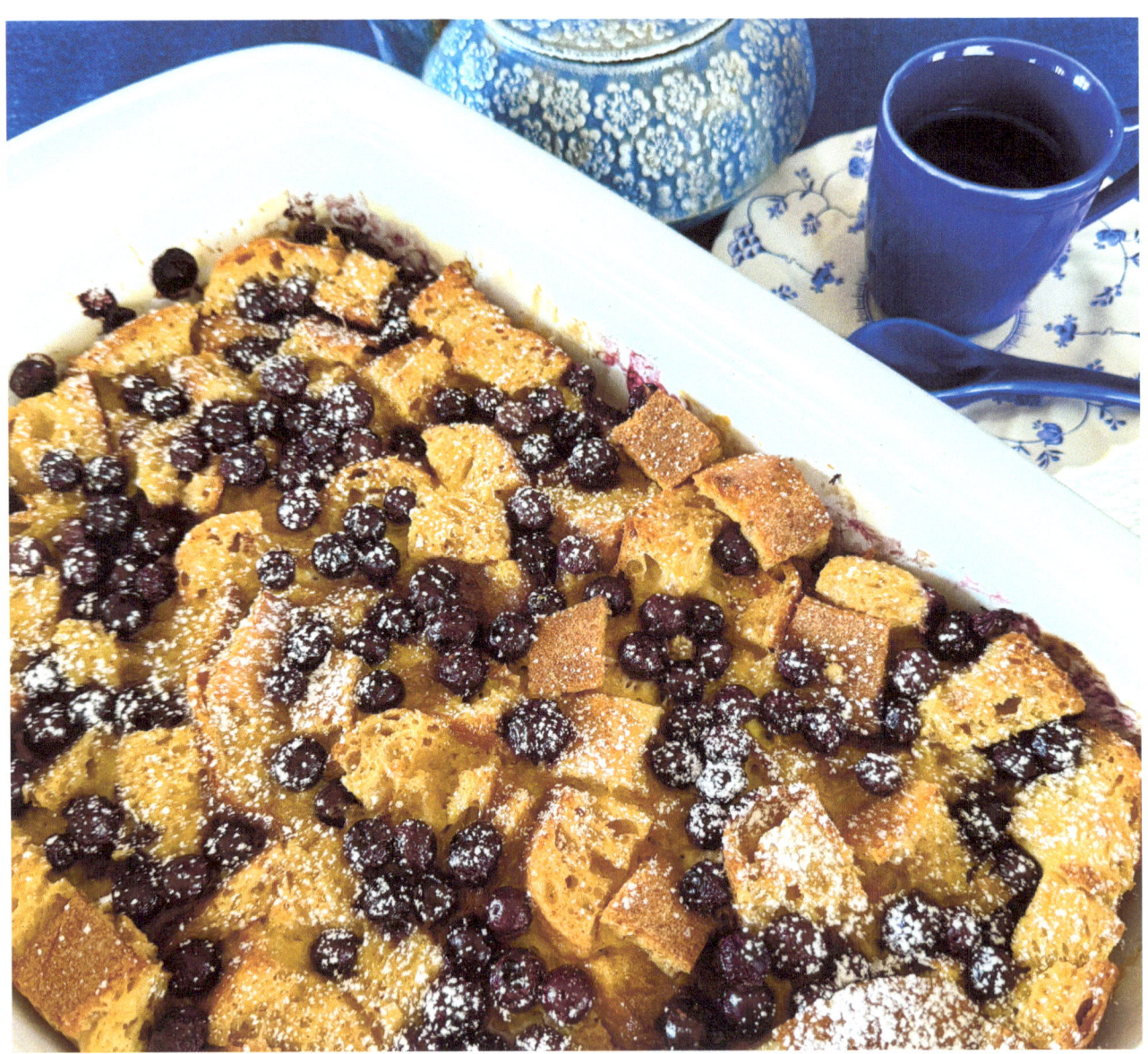

INGREDIENTS

1 lb loaf rustic French bread (slightly stale and crusty bread)

8 large eggs

2 cups (460ml) whole milk

½ cup (9 ml) heavy cream

1 tablespoon vanilla

½ teaspoon salt

½ teaspoon cinnamon

Zest and juice from 1 lemon

⅓ cup (80ml) maple syrup

2 cups (12oz) blueberries (fresh or frozen)

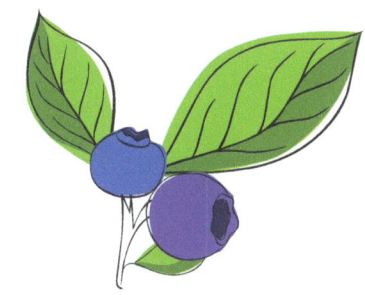

DIRECTIONS

1. **Leave the bread out uncovered overnight.** You want it to become slightly stale and crusty. If you haven't time for this, see the cooking notes below.
2. Cut the bread loaf into 1-inch cubes (to approximate 10 cups). Grease a 9 x 13-inch baking dish with butter or cooking spray and spread the bread cubes in an even layer in the baking dish.
3. Whisk the eggs slightly in a large bowl. Stir in the milk, cream, vanilla, salt, cinnamon, lemon zest, lemon juice, and maple syrup until you have a smooth batter. Pour batter evenly over the bread cubes.
4. Sprinkle the blueberries on top and gently press them into the batter.
5. Cover with plastic wrap and refrigerate for 3 to 24 hours (overnight is good).
6. When ready to bake, preheat the oven to 350°F (177°C) and let the casserole sit at room temperature for 15-20 minutes. Remove the plastic wrap and bake for 45-55 minutes, or until golden brown. The bread in the center should be moist but not liquid.
7. Serve with maple syrup and enjoy.

COOKING NOTES

- If you don't have time to leave the bread out the day before, place the bread cubes on a baking sheet and bake at 300°F for 10 minutes, or until dried.
- Using a smaller baking dish, such as a 7x11-inch dish, will give you a more "custard-like" texture, similar to a bread pudding.
- The baked casserole will freeze, tightly covered, for up to 3 months.

SUBSTITUTIONS & ADDITIONS

- For a crisper topping, sprinkle with streusel right before baking. (Recipe in Foundational chapter).
- Substitute sugar or honey for maple syrup (to your sweetness preference).
- Substitute half-and-half or almond milk for the dairy.
- Substitute sourdough or challah bread for the French bread.

Nutrition Notes (per serving): Calories 380; Protein 14g; Carbs 52g; Fat 13g; Sugar 22g

EASY — Makes 12 medium sized muffins

Blueberry Ginger Lime Muffins

I love the combination of blueberries, ginger and fresh lime. When I sold jams and syrups at the farmers' markets, this flavor profile was top of the list in popularity. I was delighted to discover that it is also the bomb in the ubiquitous blueberry muffin. Add this recipe to your catalog of easy muffin recipes and enjoy it as a healthy, delicious breakfast or portable snack.

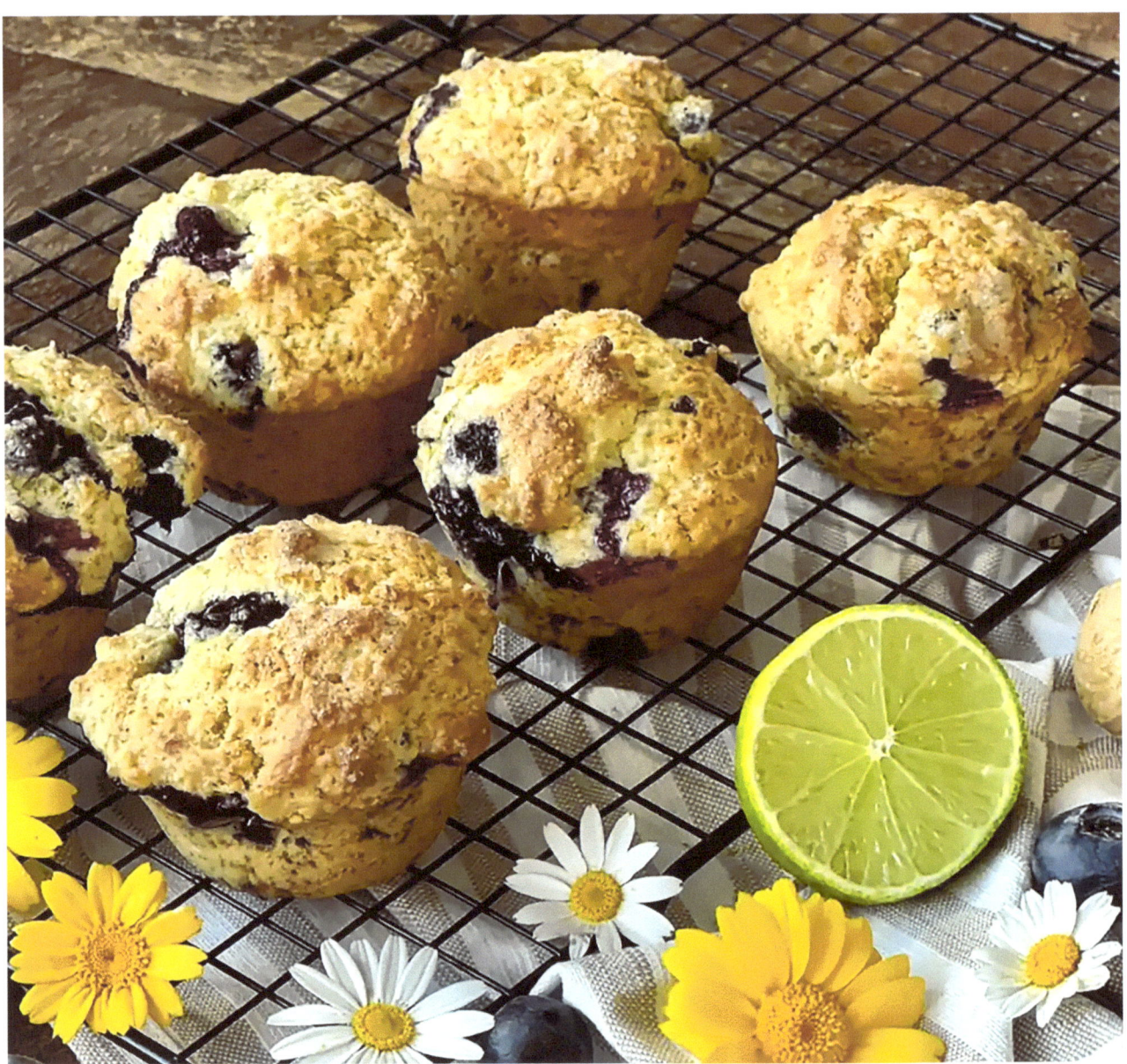

INGREDIENTS

For the Streusel Topping:

½ cup (65g) flour

½ cup (100g) sugar

¼ teaspoon salt

¼ (60g) melted butter

For the Muffins:

2 cups (250g) all-purpose flour

⅔ cup (135g) sugar

1 teaspoon baking powder

1 teaspoon baking soda

½ teaspoon kosher salt

2 cups (12oz) blueberries (unthawed frozen or fresh)

¼ cup (60g) unsalted butter

1 cup (8oz) sour cream

1 large egg, room temp.; slightly beaten

1 teaspoon lime zest

¼ cup (60ml) fresh lime juice (plus another 2 tablespoons to reserve if needed)

¼ cup (40g) crystallized ginger, minced

SUBSTITUTIONS & ADDITIONS

- Substitute lemons for limes.
- Try 1 teaspoon of cardamom and exclude the ginger.
- Buttermilk, lemon yogurt or Mexican sour cream can be used instead of sour cream.

DIRECTIONS

Preheat the oven to 400°F (204°C). Grease muffin tins (or spray with nonstick cooking spray).

For the Streusel:

1. Whisk together all streusel ingredients in a bowl and set aside to let flavors meld together.

For the Muffin Batter:

2. In a large bowl, whisk together flour, ⅔ cup sugar, baking powder, baking soda and salt. Add blueberries to the bowl and toss to coat with the flour. Set aside.

3. Melt butter (you can do this in the microwave for about 20-30 seconds) in a medium-sized bowl. To the melted butter, add sour cream, slightly beaten egg, lime zest, lime juice and the minced ginger.

4. Make a well in the center of the large bowl with the dry ingredients and add the sour cream mixture. Stir just to combine; do not overmix. If the batter seems too thick, add a little more lime juice. The batter may seem sticky—this is normal. Spoon batter into muffin cups distributing it evenly among 12 muffin cups. Sprinkle each muffin cup with the reserved streusel topping.

5. Bake for 20-25 minutes, or until muffins spring back when gently pressed with a fingertip.

6. Cool muffins for 5 minutes in the muffin tin on a wire rack. Remove muffins to rack and serve warm or cool.

Nutrition Notes: Calories 221; Protein 3g; Carbs 34g; Fat 8g; Sugar 1g

MODERATE — Makes 12 medium muffins

Bakery Style Blueberry Muffins with Cinnamon Crumb Topping

Blueberry muffins might just be the most popular muffin ever in the United States, which is why there are so many versions of them! Bakery-style refers to a domed top to the muffin, along with some sort of crumb or streusel topping to add crunch and sweetness. Although I do love dense breakfast muffins, the muffins in this recipe are light and moist, with a domed top that sparkles with a cinnamon sugar topping for the sweet crunch. And the best part? They are bursting with blueberries!

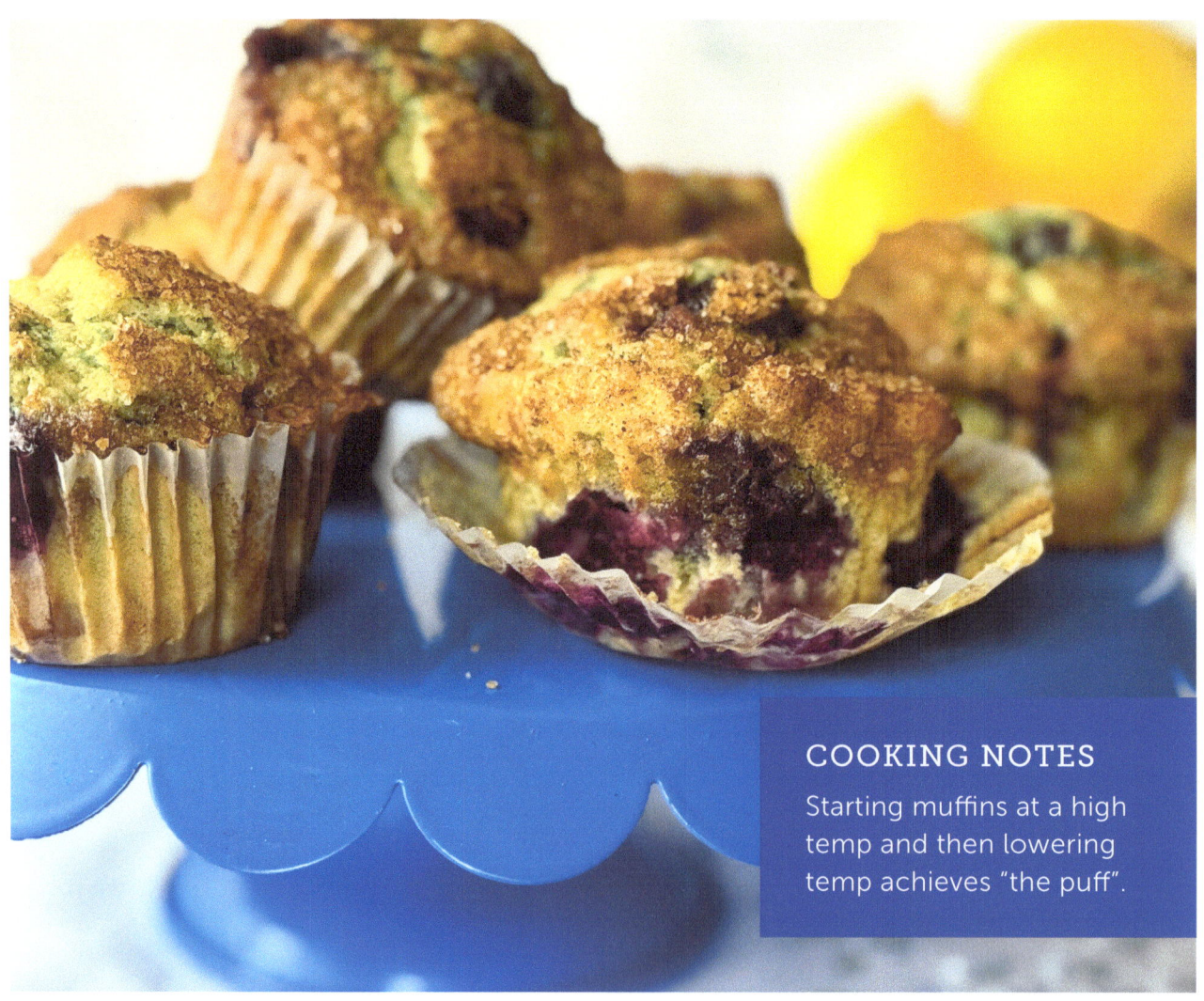

COOKING NOTES
Starting muffins at a high temp and then lowering temp achieves "the puff".

INGREDIENTS

For the Crumb Topping:

¼ cup (50g) turbinado sugar (a coarse raw sugar that can be found in the baking aisle)

Zest from ½ lemon (1-2 teaspoons)

1 teaspoon cinnamon

For the Muffin Batter:

½ cup (100g) granulated sugar

¼ cup (45g) packed brown sugar

½ cup (1 stick, 115g) unsalted butter, room temp.

2 large eggs, room temp

2 teaspoons vanilla

2 cups (240g) all-purpose flour

2 teaspoons baking powder

½ teaspoon baking soda

½ teaspoon kosher salt

½ cup (120ml) whole milk

2 cups (12oz) blueberries, frozen is best

SUBSTITUTIONS & ADDITIONS

- Substitute 1:1 gluten-free all-purpose flour replacer for the flour.
- Substitute ¼ cup sour cream and ¼ cup milk for the whole milk.
- To substitute a streusel topping instead of a crumb topping, whisk together ½ cup (65g) flour, ½ cup (100g) sugar, ¼ teaspoon salt, and ¼ cup (60g) melted butter. Set aside for ingredients to meld together.

DIRECTIONS

Preheat the oven to 425°F (218°C). Line a 12-cup muffin tray with muffin liners or generously spray muffin tin with cooking spray.

For the Crumb Topping:

1. Stir together turbinado sugar, lemon zest and cinnamon. Set aside.

For the Muffin Batter:

2. In a stand mixer with a paddle attachment (or an electric mixer), cream the sugars and the softened butter together on medium-high speed 2-3 minutes until light colored and fluffy. Scrape the sides of the mixer as you go.

3. On low speed, add the eggs, one at a time, to the mixing bowl, scraping sides between each. Add vanilla and beat until combined.

4. In a bowl, whisk together the flour, baking powder, baking soda and salt.

5. On low speed, beat in ⅓ of the flour mixture, followed by ⅓ of the milk. Repeat adding flour and milk alternately until all flour and milk have been added. Scrape the sides of the mixing bowl and beat on low for 20-30 more seconds. Batter will be thick.

6. Fold the blueberries into the batter and let it rest for 15-20 minutes (this helps create the dome top). Then using a large spoon or ice cream scoop, fill the greased muffin cups or liners all the way to the top. Sprinkle the reserved sugar topping over each muffin.

7. Bake at 425°F (218°C) for 5 minutes. Without opening the oven door, decrease the oven temperature to 350°F (177°C) and bake 15-20 minutes, or until a toothpick inserted into the middle of the muffins comes out clean.

8. Allow muffins to cool in the tin for about 5 minutes and then remove them to a wire rack to finish cooling (about 30 minutes).

Nutrition Notes (per muffin): Calories 237; Protein 4g; Carbs 36g; Fat 9g; Sugar 19g

MODERATE — Makes 8 large scones or 12 smaller scones

Blueberry Scones with Earl Grey Tea & Lavender

Classic British scones are fluffy, crumbly biscuits, meant to be paired with clotted cream and jam at a traditional "afternoon tea". American scones are more dense, often glazed or frosted, and made with many different flavor combinations—often considered a coffee shop treat.

I am a tea aficionado, but I rarely use teas in cooking. This recipe was an experiment using tea (I chose a strong Earl Grey tea) as a substitute for the cream typically found in scone recipes. I then added dried blueberries, a bit of lavender, and a topping of vanilla icing for the win.

I don't get to many formal afternoon teas, but these scones and a pot of tea at a mid-morning break from gardening make me feel ever-so-proper.

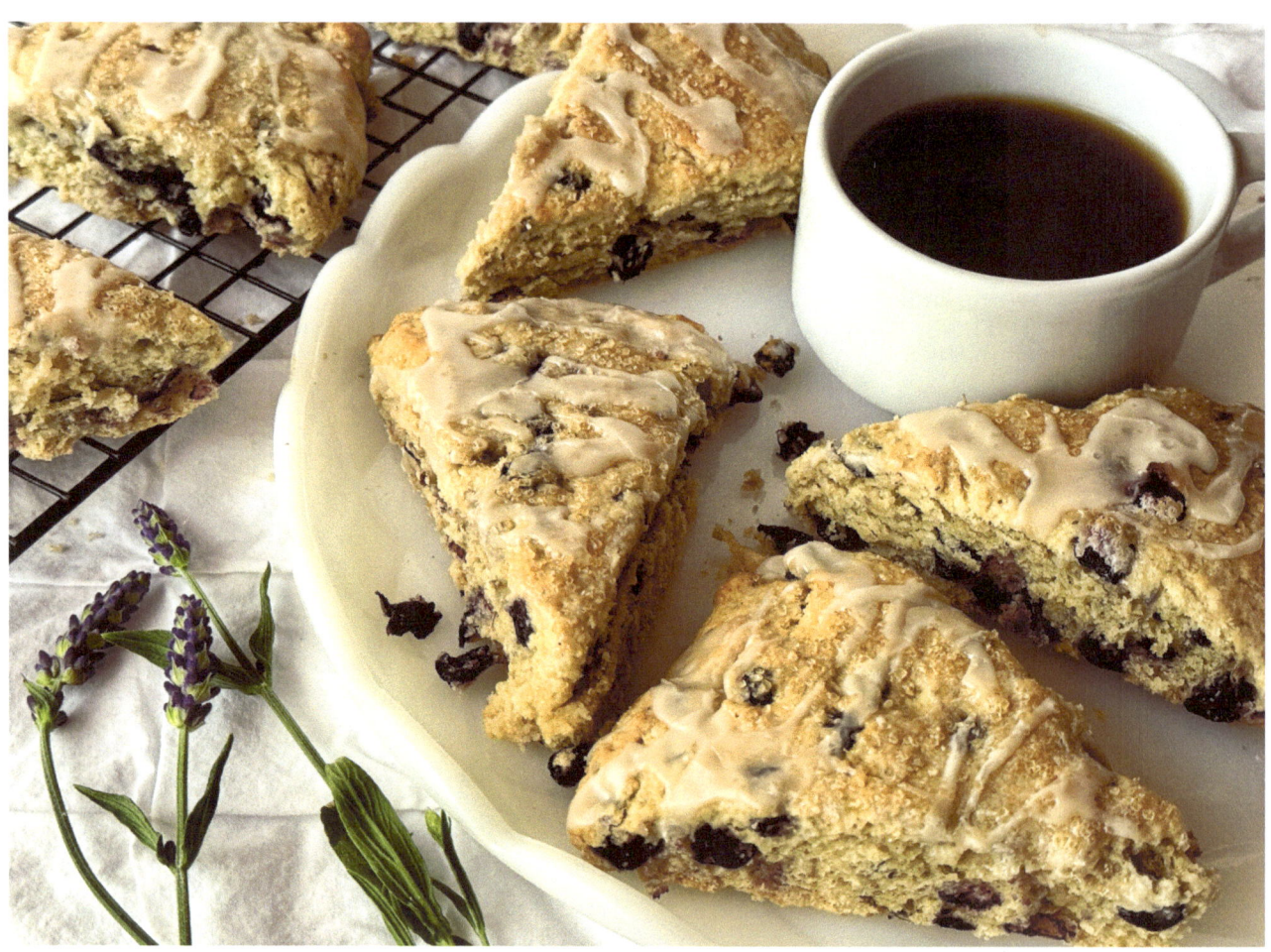

INGREDIENTS

For the Scones:

- 1 cup (90g) dried blueberries (not freeze dried)
- ¾ cup (161ml) black tea (I used Earl Grey)
- 2 ¼ cups (291g) all-purpose flour
- ⅓ cup (67g) sugar
- 1 tablespoon baking powder
- ½ teaspoon kosher salt
- ½ teaspoon ground cardamom
- 1 tablespoon dried lavender (optional)
- ½ cup (115g) unsalted butter, chilled
- 1 ½ teaspoon vanilla
- 2 tablespoons cream
- 1-2 tablespoons coarse sugar (turbinado sugar is nice)

For the Icing:

- 1 cup (133g) powdered sugar
- 1 teaspoon vanilla
- 2-3 tablespoons heavy cream

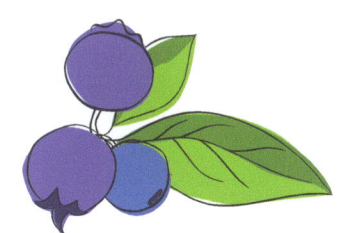

DIRECTIONS

Prepare Ingredients:

1. Rehydrate the blueberries by covering them in a liquid (warm water or juice) for at least 30 minutes. You can rehydrate with water, juice or any other liquid (juice from draining frozen blueberries is great as it adds to the blueberry flavor).
2. Make ¾ cup of tea (I used Earl Grey) and set aside to cool. I make a whole pot and just heat it up later to drink what is left.

Make Scone Dough:

3. In a large bowl, whisk together the dry ingredients (flour through dried lavender).
4. Cut the chilled butter into small pieces and add to the flour mixture. Cut the butter into the flour, until it looks like coarse crumbs with some pea-sized pieces. You can do this with a pastry cutter, 2 forks or your hands. Just move fairly fast as you don't want the butter to get warm.
5. Drain the blueberries and add them to the flour mixture, stirring to distribute evenly. Add the cooled tea and vanilla and gently mix the dough together, folding the dough rather than kneading to keep the scones tender. Do not overmix.

Nutrition Notes (for smaller scones): Calories 275; Protein 4g; Carbs 45g; Fat 9g; Sugar 24g

6. Lightly flour the counter (or a baking sheet), as well as your hands. Bring the dough together into a ball and pat out into an 8- to 9-inch round, about ¾" thick. With a sharp knife, cut into 8 wedges and place in the refrigerator to chill for a minimum of 15 minutes and up to 3 hours. I cut my wedges right on the baking sheet that I then chill and later place in the oven, but you could cut them separately and transfer to a plate. You can also freeze the dough and thaw it out when you are ready to bake.

7. Preheat the oven to 425°F (218°C). Do not remove scones from the refrigerator until the oven is fully preheated. Once the oven is ready, place scones on a baking sheet and brush with cream and sprinkle with coarse sugar. Bake for 20-25 minutes, or until light golden brown on top and around edges. Remove from oven and cool for about 5 minutes before icing.

Make the Icing:

8. While the scones are baking, whisk together the powdered sugar, vanilla and cream until there are no lumps. Drizzle the icing over the scones while they are still somewhat warm.

9. Serve with tea for the true scone experience!

COOKING NOTES

- Do not use baking soda, as it can turn the blueberries green.
- Make sure the butter is quite cold. You can even freeze it to keep it cold while cutting it in. Some cooks will grate the frozen butter using a box grater to make it easier to cut into the flour.
- Store leftover scones covered tightly at room temperature for 2 days or in the refrigerator for 5 days.
- If you want a less dense scone, use 6 tablespoons of butter instead of ½ cup (8 tablespoons).

SUBSTITUTIONS & ADDITIONS

- Any fruit can be substituted for the dried berries and it does not have to be dried. If you are using whole blueberries however, use the frozen ones (unthawed) instead of fresh for better color and distribution.
- You can soak the dried berries in brandy or an elderflower liqueur instead of water or juice for a nice addition.
- If you want a lemon flavor to your scones, substitute lemon juice for cream in the icing. Keep the acidity of the lemon juice in the icing instead of the dough however.

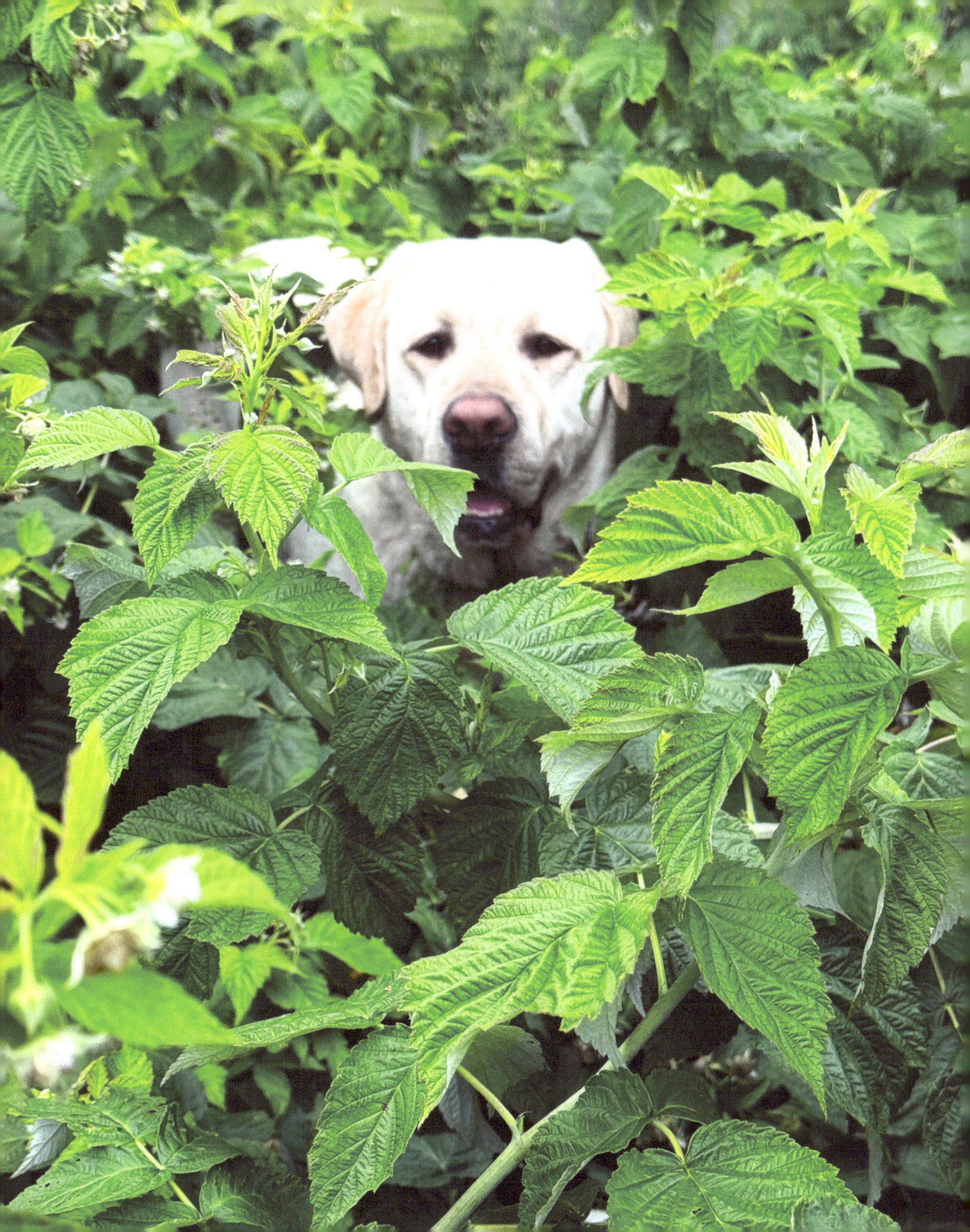

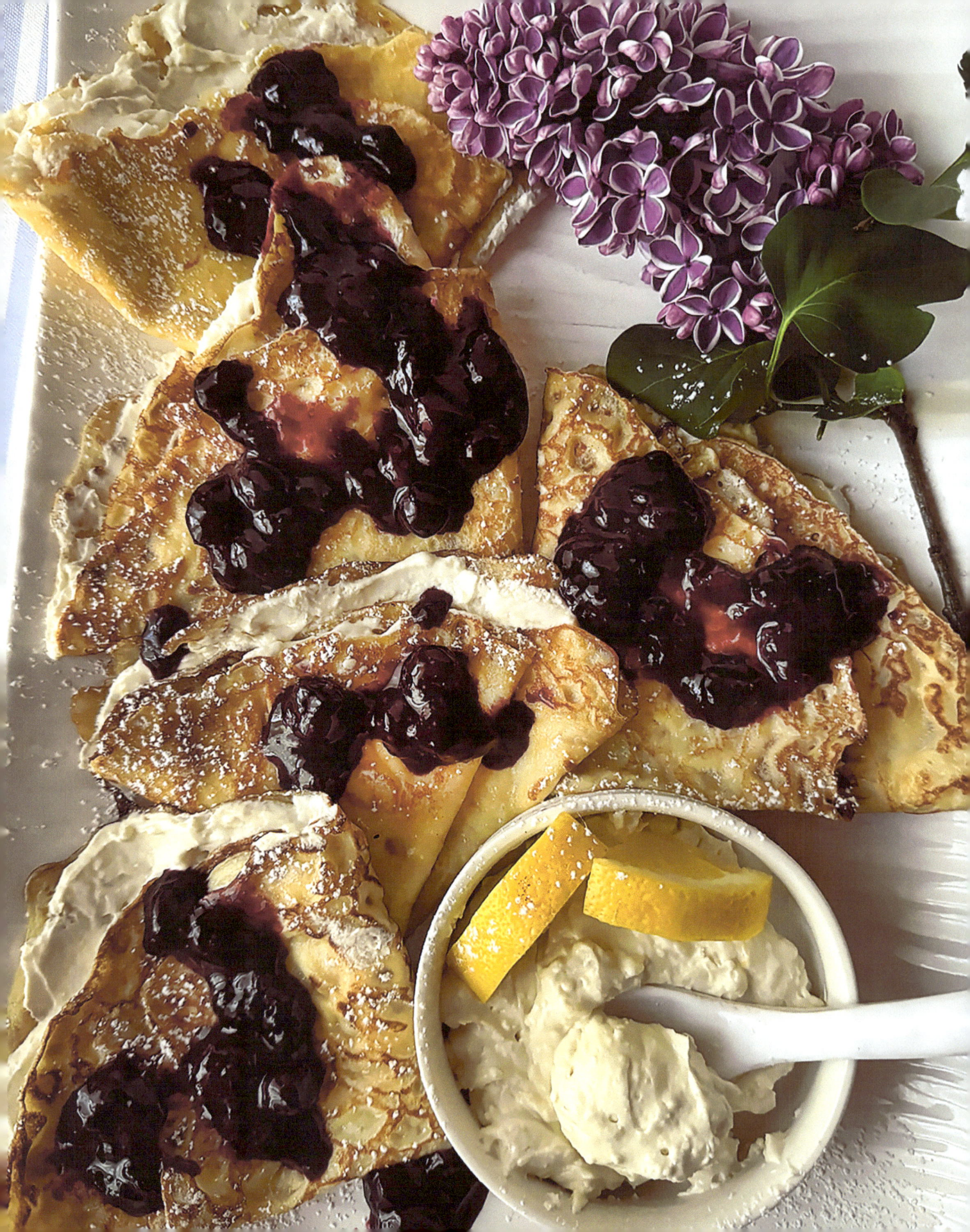

DIFFICULT — Makes 6-8 inch crêpes

Breakfast Crêpes with Ricotta Filling & Blueberry Topping

I've made these breakfast crêpes 3 times in the last month and for some reason, I got anxious each time I went to make them. If you give up on perfect circles and consider the first crepe a practice round, they become much more simple. They are quite thin and cook quickly, so make sure and have everything you need close by the crêpe pan.

This recipe is my favorite version for a breakfast crepe. They have just enough sweetness to complement the blueberries.

INGREDIENTS

For the Batter:

- 3 tablespoons (37g) unsalted butter
- 1 ½ cups (355ml) whole milk
- 1 cup (122g) all-purpose flour
- 1 tablespoon sugar
- 2 large eggs
- 1 teaspoon vanilla

For the Filling:

- 8oz (227g) ricotta cheese
- 2-4 tablespoons heavy cream
- ¼ cup powdered sugar

For the Compote:

- 2 tablespoons sugar
- ¼ cup water
- 1 tablespoon cornstarch
- 1 tablespoon lemon zest
- ½ teaspoon vanilla
- 2 cups (12oz) blueberries (fresh or frozen)

DIRECTIONS

Make the Batter:

1. Melt the butter in a microwave and set aside to cool slightly.
2. In a blender, combine milk, flour, sugar, eggs, vanilla and the cooled softened butter. Blend until thoroughly combined (about 20-30 seconds), scraping flour from bottom of blender if it settles there. Place the blender, with the cover on, in the refrigerator for 30 minutes or more.

Make the Filling:

3. In a bowl, whisk together the ricotta, the cream and the sugar until thoroughly combined with no lumps left. Refrigerate, covered, until ready to use.

Make the Compote:

4. In a medium saucepan over medium-high heat, whisk together the sugar, water, cornstarch, lemon zest and vanilla. Cook 1-2 minutes until sugar and cornstarch are dissolved. Add the blueberries and bring everything to a boil. Reduce heat and cook, stirring constantly until sauce is slightly

Nutrition (includes filling & topping): Calories 356; Protein 11g; Carbs 43g; Fat 16g; Sugar 24g

thickened (about 2 minutes or more for a thicker sauce).

Make the Crêpes:

5. Assemble everything you will need next to your stovetop: a crêpe pan or an 8-inch skillet with no high sides, about 4 tablespoons of butter, the bowl of batter, the wax paper or parchment paper if stacking crêpes, paper towels or pastry brush for spreading butter, a ¼ cup measuring cup for ladling out the crêpes, and a wooden crêpe spreader if available.

6. Place the crêpe pan over medium-high heat and use a paper towel or pastry brush to coat the bottom of the pan with butter. If butter doesn't sizzle, let it get a little hotter before adding the batter.

7. Pour ¼ cup of batter into the middle of the pan and immediately pick up the pan and swirl it around to get the batter to form an even layer on the bottom of the pan (a circle). If you have a crêpe spreader, use it to form a thin circle of batter (this takes a little practice).

8. When crêpe has browned slightly on the bottom or around the edges (about 1 minute), slip a thin spatula under it and flip. It is easier to flip if you keep it fairly close to the pan and forgo the theatrics. Cook the second side briefly, just enough to set the batter.

9. Slide the crêpe from the pan onto a sheet of wax paper or parchment paper on a plate. Regrease the pan with more butter and repeat the steps, placing the wax paper between each crêpe as you stack them on the plate. At this point you can place the stack in a plastic bag and store it in the refrigerator for a few days or in the freezer for a few months.

Assemble and Fold the Crêpes:

10. There are many ways to fill and fold a crêpe. I have included photo collages of the four simplest methods on the following page. Choose one of these folding methods, spread a couple of tablespoons of ricotta filling in each one, and top with the blueberry compote.

SUBSTITUTIONS & ADDITIONS

- Substitute half milk and half water for a thinner, more delicate crêpe.
- Substitute ½ cup beer and ½ cup milk for a crispier texture.
- Crêpes are a blank canvas for fillings and toppings. The ricotta can easily be replaced with cream cheese or mascarpone.
- The compote works well with strawberries or other small berries.

COOKING NOTES

- Make sure to chill the batter for 30-60 minutes before making the crêpes. It gives the flour time to fully hydrate.
- Use a paper towel to spread a small piece of butter around the pan between each crêpe.
- Try to twirl the batter as thinly as you can. This will result in a better texture and the crispy edges.
- If you are making crêpes for a crowd, preheat the oven to 200°F (93°C) and keep them warm on a heat-proof platter in the oven.

3 Easy Ways to Fold Crepes

THE ENVELOPE FOLD

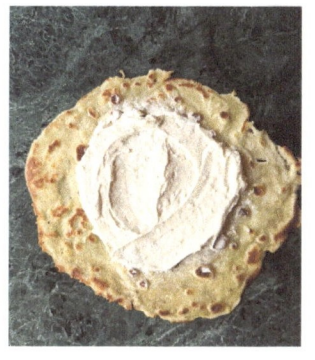 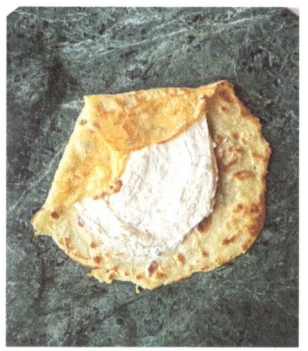 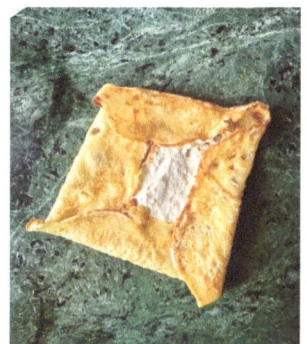 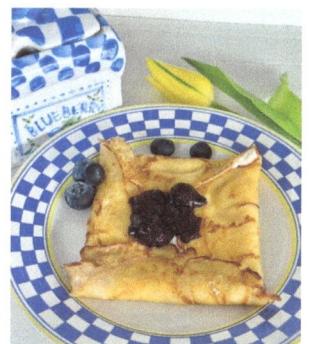

THE OPEN ROLL

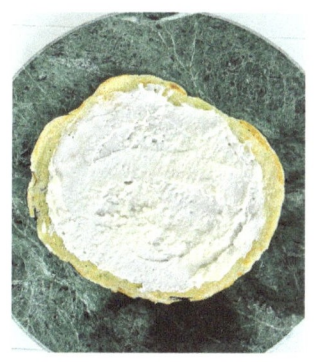 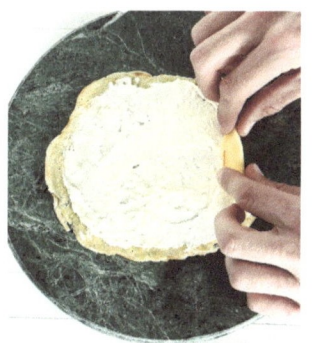 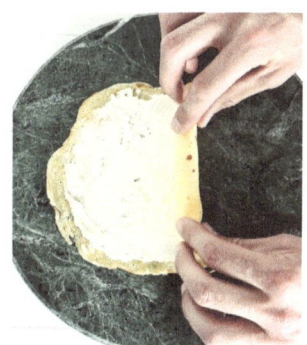 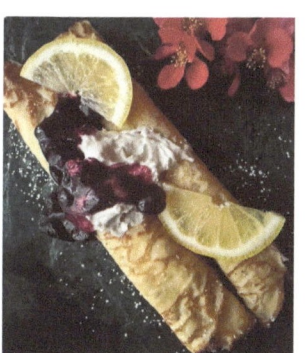

THE ¼ TRIANGLE FOLD

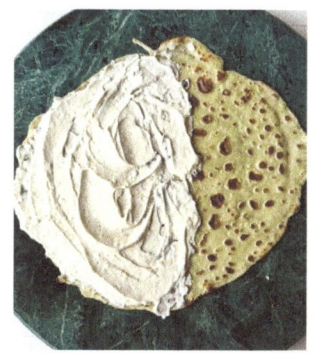 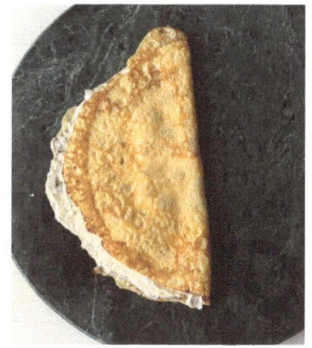 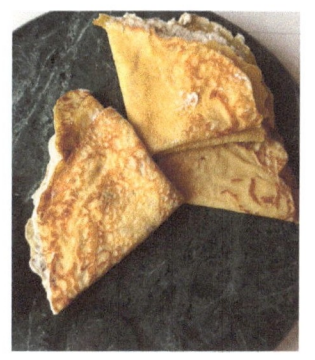 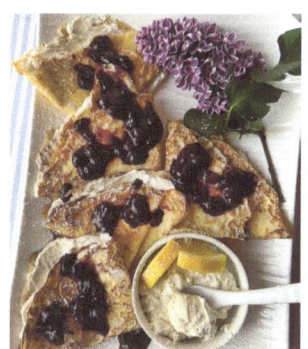

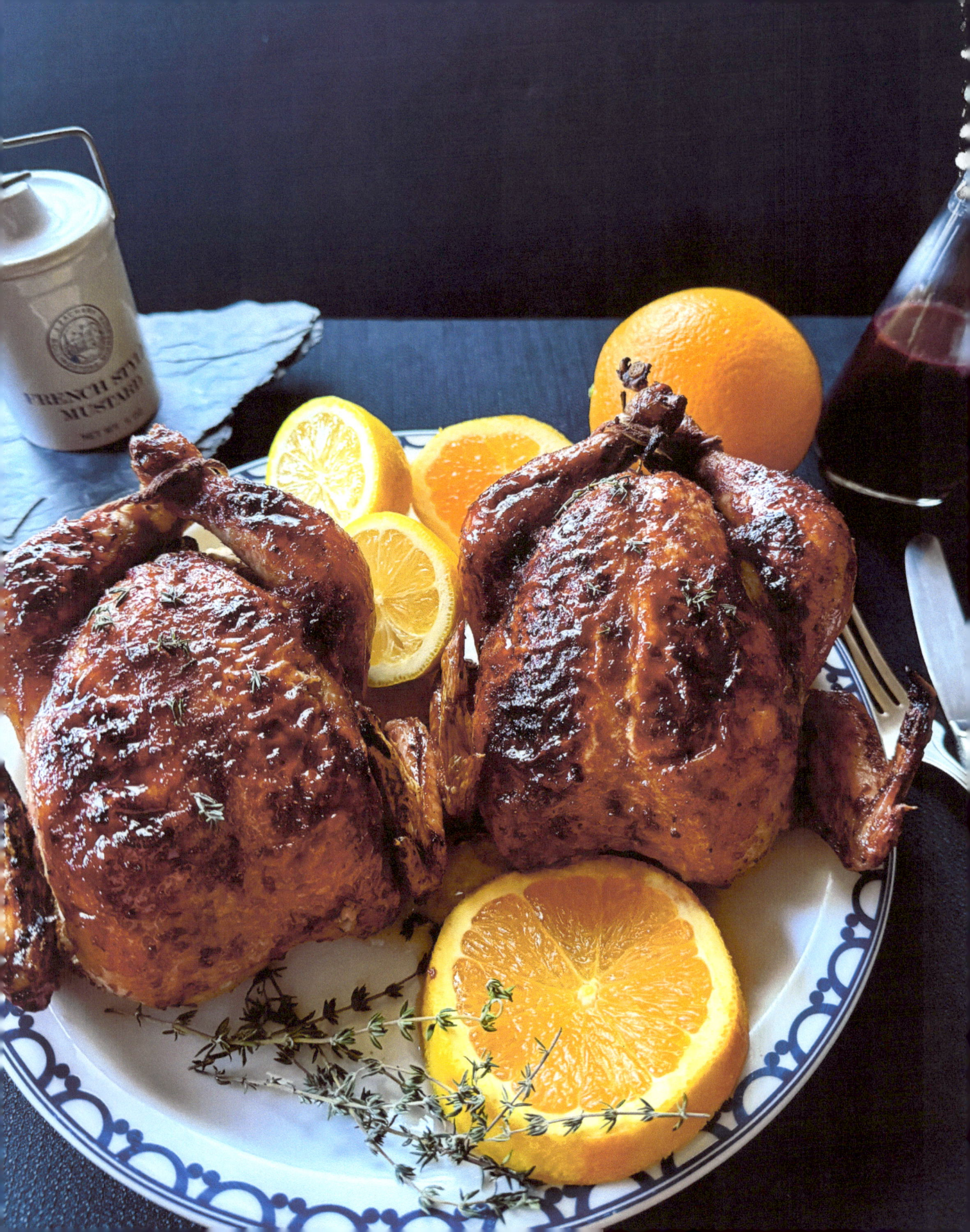

SAVORY MAIN DISHES

- Chicken & Blueberry Dinner Salad
- Easy Pizza with Prosciutto, Goat Cheese & Pickled Blueberries
- Vegetarian Squash & Brown Rice Salad with Chipotle Dressing
- Salmon & Blueberry-Corn Salsa
- Pork Chops with Blueberry BBQ Sauce
- Blueberry-Glazed Baby Back Ribs
- Cornish Game Hens with Blueberry Cumberland Sauce
- Blueberry BBQ Bacon Cheeseburger

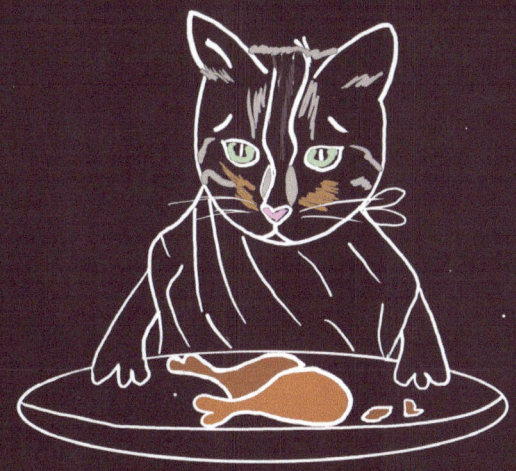

EASY — Serves 4 (large dinner plates) — Allow 1 hour for chicken to marinate

Chicken & Blueberry Dinner Salad

The problem with most dinner salads? They're either boring or they try too hard. This one hits that sweet spot where everything just works. The blueberries add natural sweetness that pairs beautifully with the tangy vinaigrette, while the protein-rich chicken keeps it from feeling like rabbit food. It's a fresh, summery meal that actually makes you excited about eating salad for dinner.

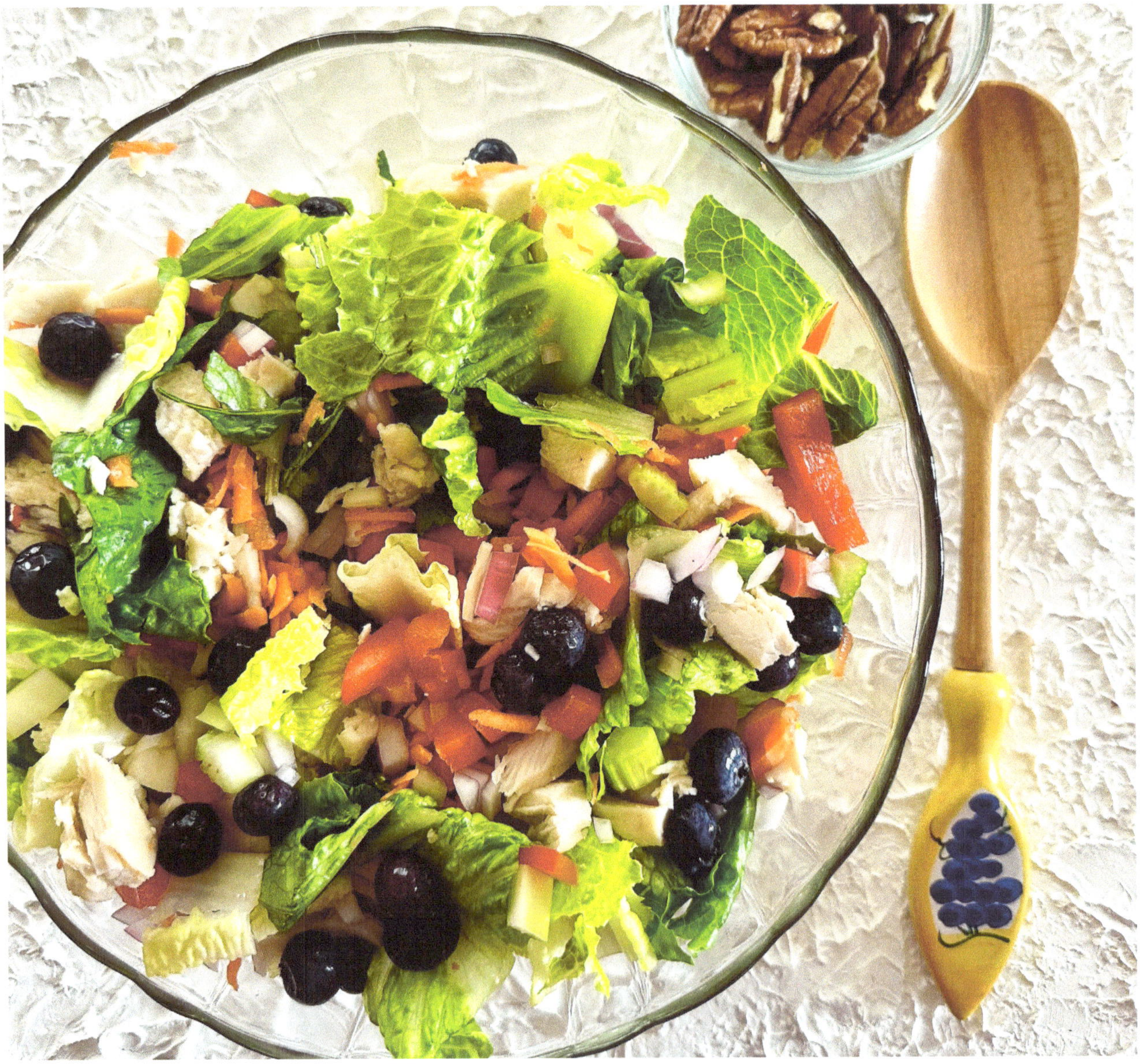

INGREDIENTS

1 lb boneless, skinless chicken breasts

6 tablespoons olive oil (for dressing/marinade)

⅓ cup (80 ml) white wine vinegar

3-4 cloves garlic, minced

4 teaspoons lemon juice

¼ teaspoon kosher salt

1 tablespoon olive oil (for cooking)

2 carrots, shredded

2 celery ribs, chopped

½ cup (75 g) chopped onion (optional)

½ cup (75 g) chopped red bell pepper

4 cups torn salad greens

2 cups (12 oz) fresh blueberries

SUBSTITUTIONS & ADDITIONS

- You can substitute pre-cooked rotisserie chicken for the chicken breasts.
- Add or substitute tomatoes for the peppers.
- Substitute your favorite salad dressing for the vinaigrette.
- Strawberries work well as a substitute for blueberries.

COOKING NOTES

- This recipe is really best with fresh berries. Frozen can be used in a pinch, but make sure they are thawed and thoroughly dried.
- Internal temperature is the most reliable doneness test—invest in an instant-read thermometer for accuracy.

DIRECTIONS

1. In a small bowl, whisk together the 6 tablespoons olive oil, vinegar, garlic, lemon juice, and salt. Pour half of the dressing in a bowl and set aside for the salad dressing. Pour the remaining half into a large ziplock bag, add the chicken breasts, and marinate for about an hour.

2. After about an hour, remove the chicken from the marinade and discard the used marinade. Pat the chicken dry with paper towels, and pound the chicken breasts thin with something heavy and flat (like the bottom of a wide jar or a mallet). Season with salt and pepper to taste.

3. Heat 1 tablespoon olive oil in a large skillet over medium-high heat. Add the chicken breasts and reduce the heat to medium (don't crowd the breasts in the pan).

4. Cook for 2-3 minutes over medium to achieve a light golden sear and then flip. Reduce heat to low and cover the pan. Cook, covered, on low for 10 minutes without lifting the lid. Then turn off the heat and let the skillet sit (keeping it covered) for another 10 minutes.

5. Uncover and check to make sure chicken is done (no pink in the middle of the breasts). Chicken should be 165°F. Set aside breasts to cool to room temperature.

For the Salad:

1. While the chicken is cooking and then cooling (Step 4 above), shred the carrots and chop the celery, onion, and pepper. Tear the lettuce into bite-size pieces

2. After the chicken has cooled, cut or tear it into bite-size pieces.

3. In a large bowl, toss all ingredients except blueberries with the reserved dressing. Add the blueberries and gently toss to combine.

Nutrition Notes (per serving): Calories 234; Protein 26g; Carbs 18g; Fat 7; Sugar 10g

🥄 EASY — Makes a 10 x 13-inch pizza (about 6 servings)

Easy Pizza with Prosciutto, Goat Cheese & Pickled Blueberries

Blueberry season in the Midwest is short but intense, and there is a rush to make all those delightful cobblers and muffins while the berries are still fresh. This recipe takes blueberries in a different direction, where the sweetness of the berry plays against salty prosciutto and creamy goat cheese. The fresh greens add a peppery bite that ties it all together, giving you a savory treat for the blue jewel..

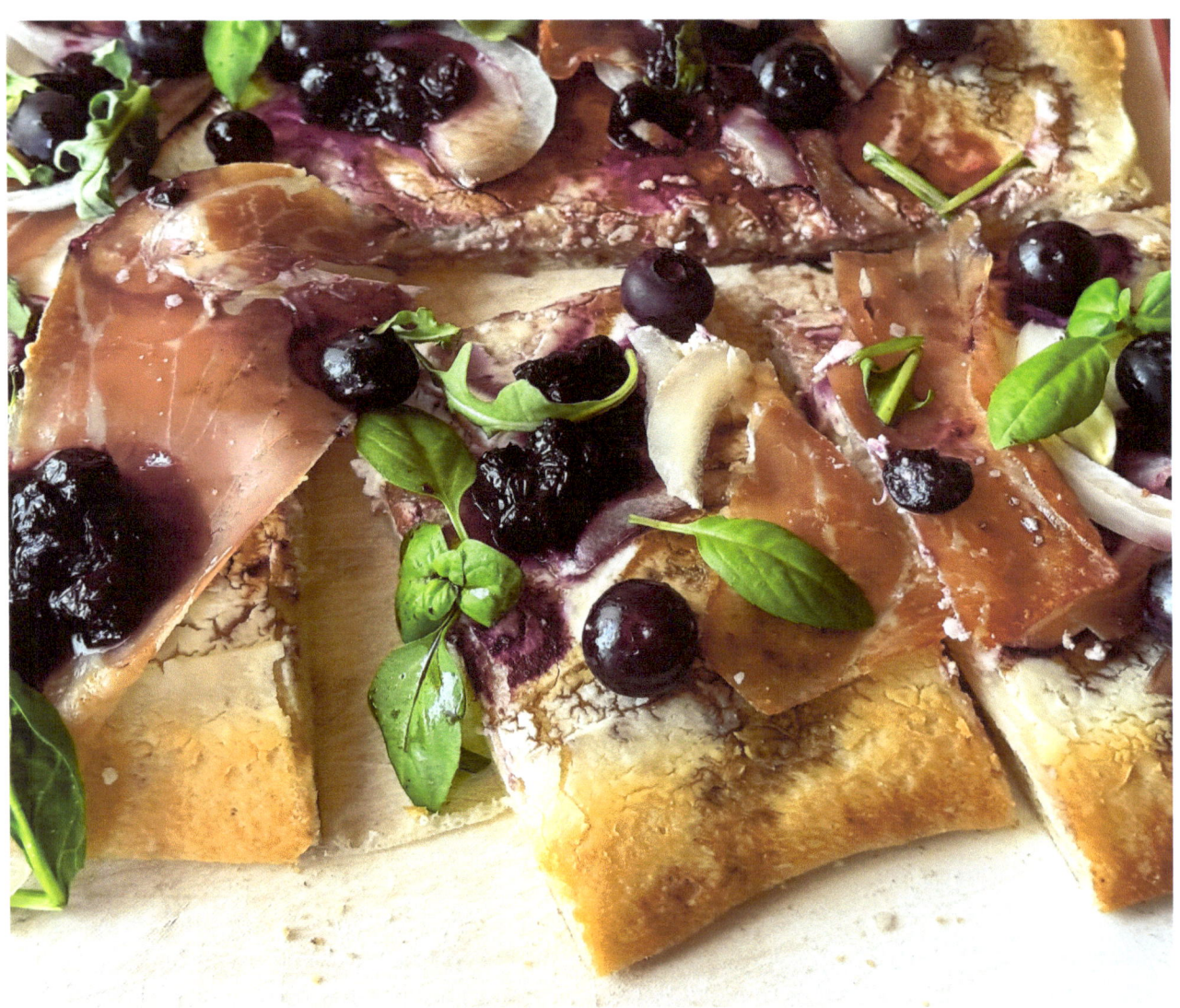

INGREDIENTS

1 package (about 14 oz) store-bought pizza dough (I used Pillsbury Pizza Crust), room temp.

1 tablespoon olive oil

6 oz goat cheese, softened

4 oz (115 g) sliced purple onion

4 oz (115 g) sliced prosciutto

2/3 cup (4 oz) blueberries; you can use fresh or frozen blueberries. I used pickled blueberries to add some tang (recipe for pickled blueberries is in the foundational recipes chapter)

1 cup spinach

½ cup arugula

¼ cup basil leaves

1 tablespoon balsamic vinegar

COOKING NOTES

- Prosciutto is salty so do not add salt to the crust.
- I used Pillsbury crust because it was available at my local store. Just follow the directions on the package for bake times if you use a different brand of pizza (or flatbread) dough.

DIRECTIONS

1. Preheat the oven to 400°F (204°C).

Prebake the Dough:

2. On a piece of parchment paper, roll out the store-bought pizza dough into the shape of a 10 x 13 rectangle (lightly flour the rolling pin to avoid sticking). Transfer the parchment paper to a large sheet pan and brush the dough with a tablespoon of olive oil. When the oven has preheated, prebake the dough for about 8 minutes, or until light golden brown.

3. While dough is baking, slice the onions thinly and crumble the goat cheese. Have all toppings ready before starting assembly.

Assemble & Bake the Pizza:

4. Remove the pre-baked crust from the oven and distribute the goat cheese over the crust. Once the crumbles of goat cheese are distributed, use a spatula to spread it out evenly over the crust. Then distribute the prosciutto and sliced onions over the goat cheese, covering the pizza.

5. Bake pizza 5-6 minutes, or until cheese is soft and prosciutto is a little crisp. Remove from oven and top with the blueberries and spinach. Bake for another 3-4 minutes.

6. Remove from the oven and top with the basil and arugula. Drizzle with the balsamic vinegar and let it rest for a few minutes. Cut into squares and serve warm.

Nutrition Notes (per slice): Calories 353; Protein 19g; Carbs 37g; Fat 17g; Sugar 4g

MODERATE — Makes 6 servings (about 1 cup each)

Vegetarian Squash & Brown Rice Salad with Chipotle Dressing

The challenge with vegetarian dinners is making them feel substantial enough to satisfy everyone at the table. This pilaf solves that problem by combining hearty brown rice with roasted butternut squash and a bold chipotle dressing that brings everything together. The blueberries add unexpected bursts of sweetness that balance the smoky heat, while the pepitas give it the crunch that makes each bite interesting.

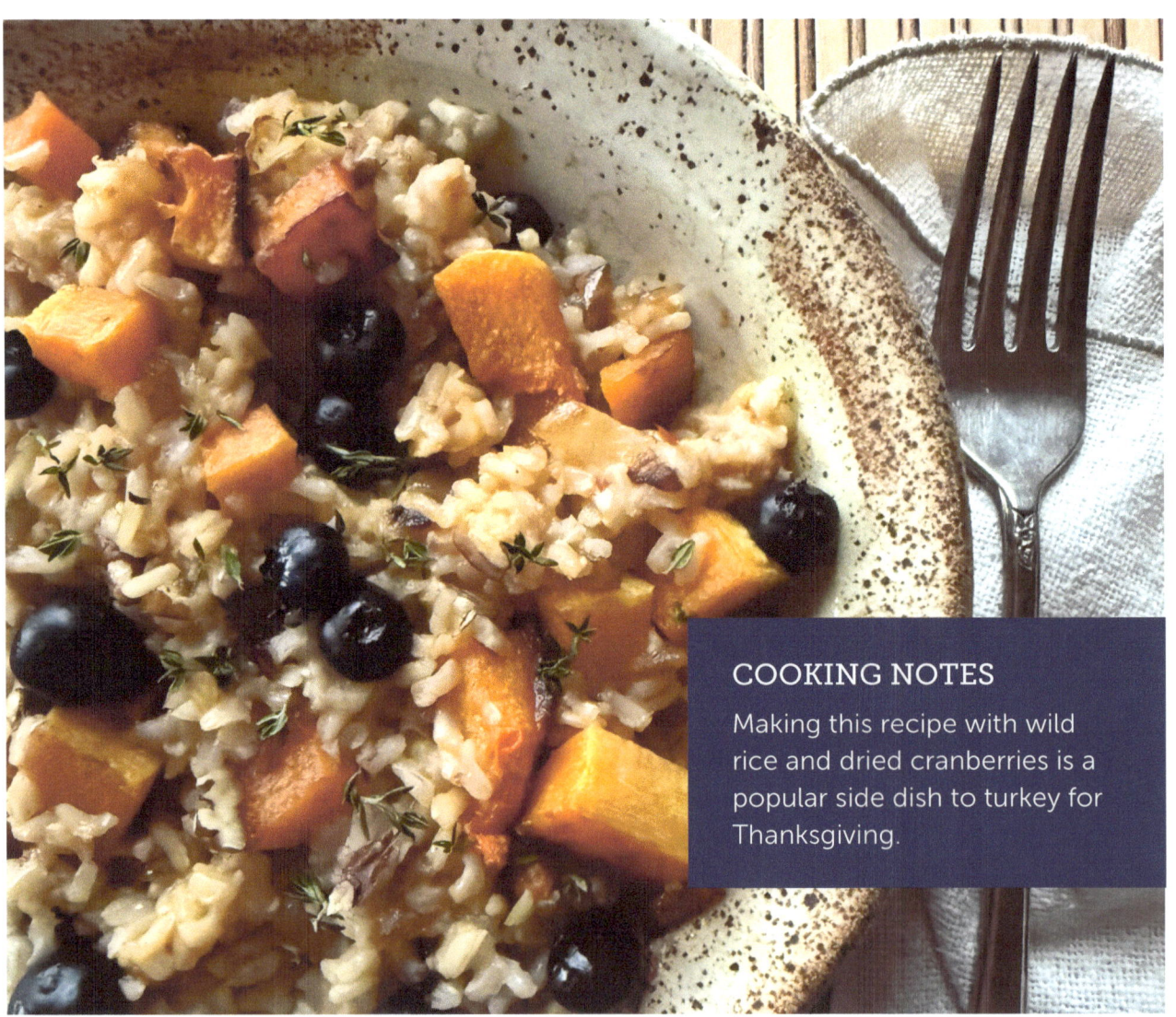

COOKING NOTES

Making this recipe with wild rice and dried cranberries is a popular side dish to turkey for Thanksgiving.

INGREDIENTS

For the Pilaf:

1 ½ cups (270 g) brown rice

3 ½ cups (840 ml) water

½ teaspoon kosher salt

5 cups (1 ½ lb/680 g) peeled, chopped butternut squash (can use pre-cut squash)

2 tablespoons olive oil (divided)

1 teaspoon kosher salt

1 medium onion (about 150 g), chopped

2 cloves garlic, peeled & minced

1 cup (6 oz) blueberries

½ cup pepitas (pumpkin seeds)

For the Chipotle Dressing:

6 tablespoons lemon juice

2 tablespoons honey

½ cup (120 ml) olive oil

1-2 chiles from chile adobo can

1 tablespoon adobo sauce

2 cloves garlic, peeled and minced

½ teaspoon kosher salt

SUBSTITUTIONS & ADDITIONS

- Substitute pecans or walnuts for the pepitas.
- Substitute wild rice for the brown rice and make according to package directions.
- Substitute store-bought cubed squash if you don't want to peel and de-seed your own.
- Substitute your favorite citrus dressing instead of the chipotle dressing.

DIRECTIONS

1. Preheat oven to 400°F (204°C).
2. Add the rice, water and salt to a large saucepan, stir, and bring to a boil over medium high heat. Once boiling, reduce the heat to low, cover the pot, and simmer rice about 40 minutes. Check occasionally to make sure it isn't starting to burn, adding a little water if needed. Remove from burner and let it rest 5-10 minutes.
3. While rice is cooking, peel and de-seed squash. To deseed the squash, cut in half lengthwise and use a sturdy spoon to scrape out the seeds and pulp from the center hollow. Cut the peeled, de-seeded squash into ½ to ¾ inch cubes (or bite size pieces).
4. Spread squash pieces on a baking sheet and drizzle with 1 tablespoon olive oil and sprinkle with salt. Using your hands, toss the squash pieces together to coat with the oil and salt.
5. Bake squash pieces for 20 minutes, toss them to brown the other side, and bake for 15 more minutes. Watch them during the last 15 minutes to prevent burning.
6. In a large skillet heat the remaining 1 tablespoon olive oil over medium heat. Sauté the chopped onion for 5-10 minutes or until softened and caramelized. Stir in the minced garlic and cook for 30 seconds. Add the cooked rice to the skillet and stir to combine.

For the chipotle dressing:

7. Add all ingredients to a blender and blend until smooth.
8. Scrape the rice and onion mixture into a large serving bowl and add some of the chipotle dressing and stir to combine (I used about ½ of the dressing).
9. Fold in the roasted squash, top with blueberries and pepitas. Serve warm or cold.

Nutrition Notes (per serving): Calories 308; Protein 7 g; Carbs 63 g; Fat 5 g; Sugar 12 g

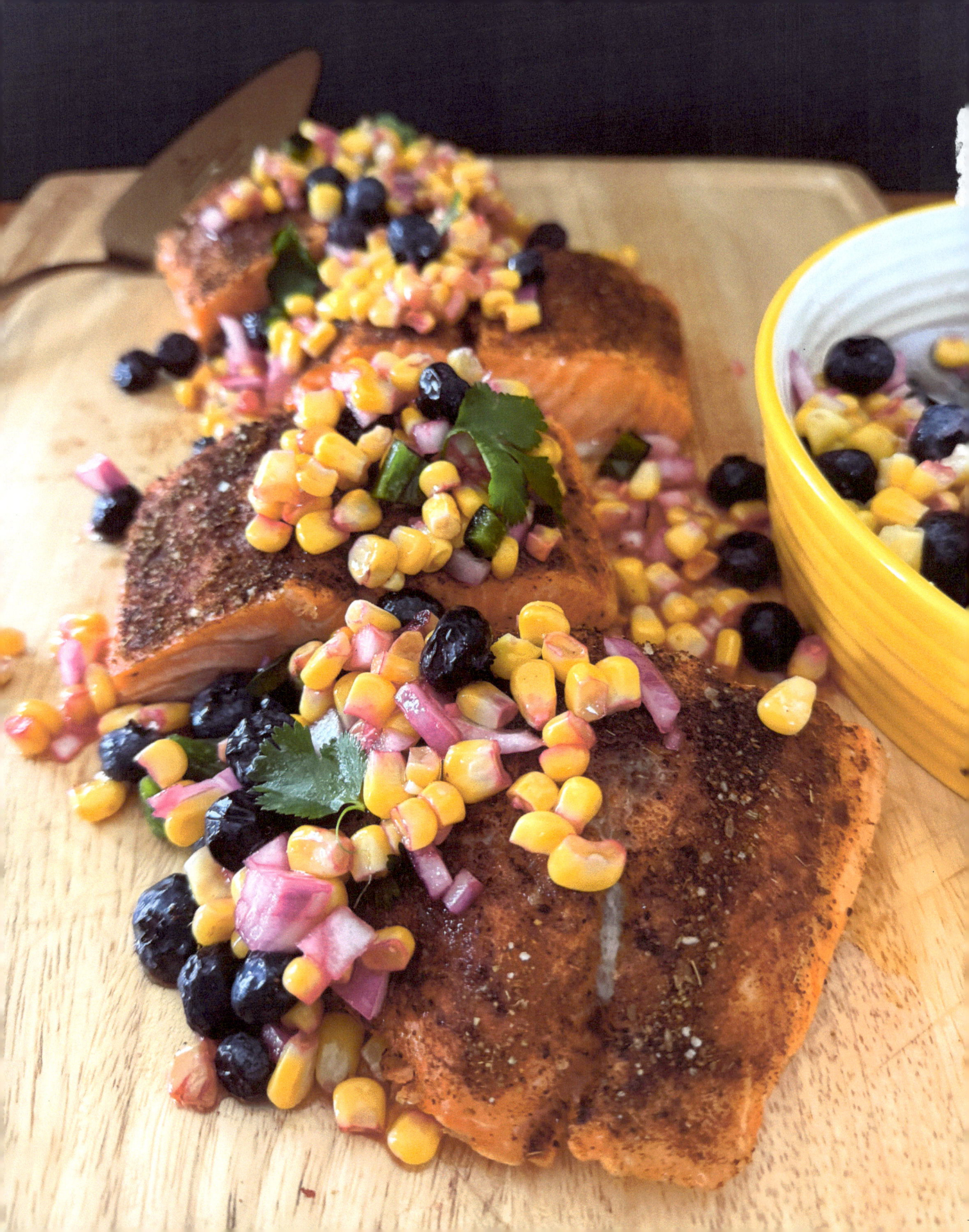

MODERATE — Makes 6 6-oz filets

Salmon & Blueberry-Corn Salsa

Salmon can be tricky--cook it plain and it's boring, whereas many of the "flavorful" recipes I've tried end up masking the essence of the fish. This recipe finds the sweet spot by using a chile spice rub and a blueberry corn salsa, enhancing the flavor of the salmon rather than overwhelming it.

INGREDIENTS

For the Salmon:

- 6 6-oz salmon filets (36 oz total)
- 2 teaspoons powdered chipotle peppers
- 1 teaspoon ground cumin
- ½ teaspoon kosher salt
- ½ teaspoon ground coriander
- 1 tablespoon brown sugar

For the Dressing:

- 4 tablespoons white wine vinegar
- 2 teaspoons lemon juice
- 6 tablespoons olive oil

For the Dressing:

- 2 cups (12oz) fresh blueberries
- 3 cups (450 g) corn kernels, fresh or defrosted frozen
- ⅓ cup (50 g) diced purple onion
- ¼ cup (40 g) diced poblano pepper
- ½ teaspoon kosher salt
- ¼ cup cilantro or basil leaves

DIRECTIONS

1. Preheat the oven to 400°F (204°C).
2. In a small bowl, whisk together the chipotle spice, cumin, salt, coriander, and brown sugar for the salmon spice blend.
3. Place salmon filets on a baking sheet and evenly divide the spice blend over each filet, rubbing it in with your hands.
4. Roast salmon in the oven for 10-12 minutes, or until it flakes easily with a fork and is opaque throughout the flesh.
5. While the salmon is roasting, make the corn salsa. In a small bowl whisk together the vinegar, lemon juice, and olive oil. Set aside and let the flavors meld together.
6. In a large bowl combine the blueberries, corn kernels, diced onion, diced poblano pepper and salt.
7. Pour the dressing over the salsa mixture, add the cilantro or basil and gently toss everything together to combine.
8. When salmon is done, remove from oven. Spoon some of the blueberry corn salsa over the top of the salmon and serve the remaining salsa on the side.

SUBSTITUTIONS & ADDITIONS

- Jalapeño peppers can be substituted for the poblano if you like it spicier
- Champagne vinegar or sherry vinegar are nice substitutes for the white wine vinegar.

Nutrition Notes (per serving): Calories 274; Protein 34g; Carbs 8g; Fat 11g; Sugar 5g

MODERATE — Makes 3 large bone-in chops

Pork Chops with Blueberry BBQ Sauce

Pork chops have a bad-boy reputation. They are either dry as a bone or dangerously undercooked. This recipe fixes both problems by using a foolproof sear-and-braise technique with a homemade blueberry BBQ sauce. The BBQ sauce keeps the chops moist while adding layers of smoky, fruity flavor, transforming them into something that tastes like a summer barbecue, even when you're cooking indoors.

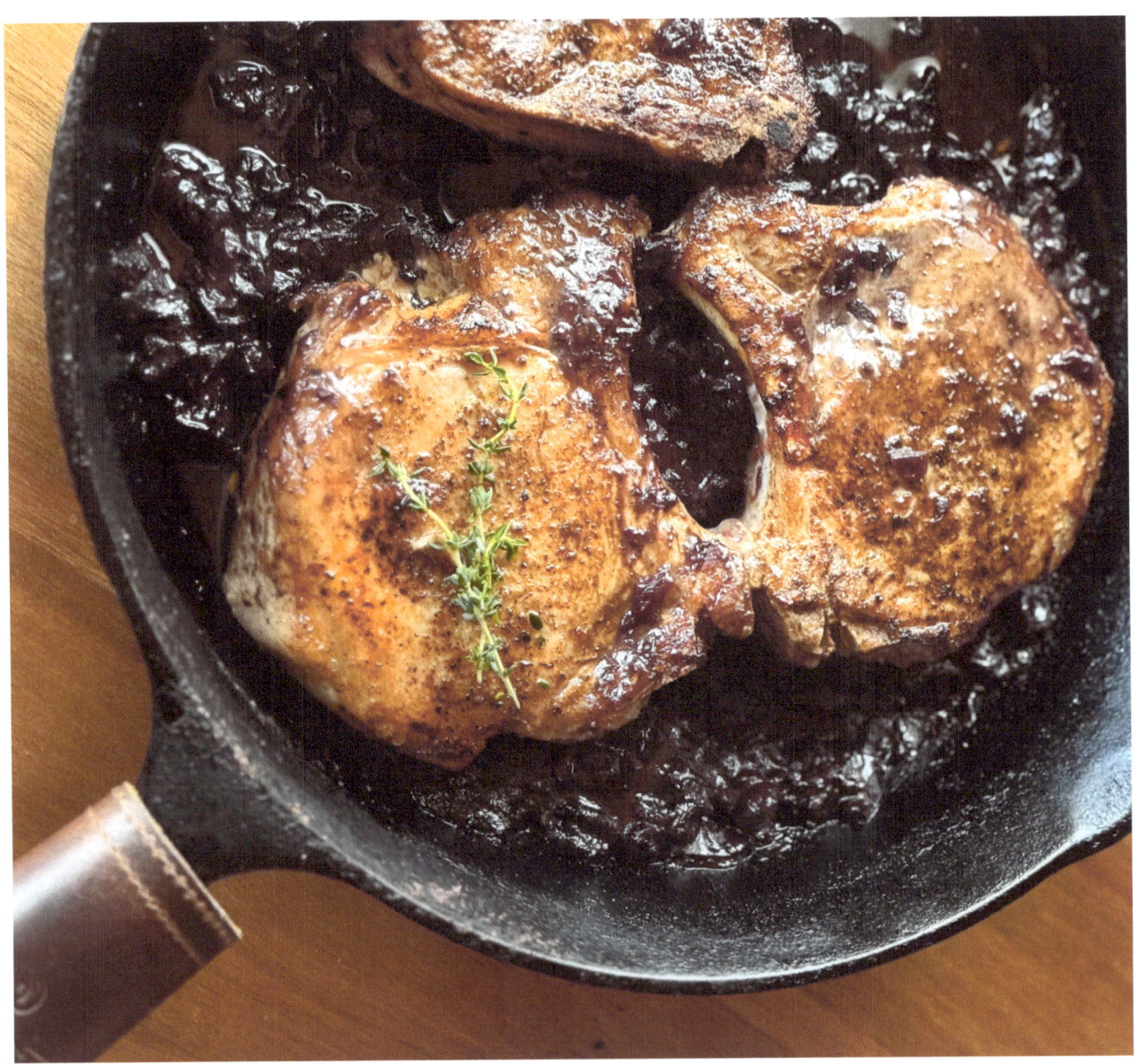

INGREDIENTS

For the Blueberry BBQ Sauce

- ½ teaspoon hot sauce (I use Cholula)
- ½ teaspoon liquid smoke
- ½ cup (3.5 oz) ketchup
- ¼ cup (60 ml) balsamic vinegar
- 3-4 tablespoons brown sugar (packed)
- 3 tablespoons Dijon mustard
- ⅛ teaspoon ground allspice
- 1 tablespoon oil
- ½ medium onion, chopped (75 g)
- 3 cloves garlic, minced
- ⅓ cup (80 ml) bourbon (optional)
- 3 cups (18 oz) blueberries (fresh or frozen)
- ½ teaspoon kosher salt

For the Pork Chop:

- 3 tablespoons unsalted butter
- Salt & pepper (or use your favorite rub)
- 3 large (14-16 oz) bone-in pork chops (1 ½ inch thick), room temperature
- ½ cup blueberry BBQ sauce (from above)

COOKING NOTES

- Cooking time can vary based on the thickness of the pork chops.
- The chops should have a slight resistance when you press on them with your finger, but not feel hard and solid.
- Boneless chops have less flavor than bone-in. I don't trim the fat, as the fat keeps them from drying out.
- It is important to not overcook the chops. They will continue to rise 5-7 degrees as they rest.

DIRECTIONS

Make the Blueberry Sauce:

1. In a bowl, mix together the first seven ingredients (hot sauce through allspice). Set aside.
2. Heat oil over medium-high in a large skillet, add chopped onions, and sauté for about 5 minutes until soft. Add garlic to the skillet and cook briefly (30 seconds).
3. Add bourbon (if using) and bring to a low boil for about 3 minutes. Add the blueberries and the reserved sauce mixture, stir, and return to a boil. Add the salt, lower the heat and simmer for about 20 minutes, or until thickened to your preference. Remove from heat and set aside.

Make the Pork Chops:

4. Add butter to a large skillet and melt over medium-high heat until bubbly. It's OK if it turns brown, but don't let it burn.
5. Season chops with salt and pepper (or your favorite spice rub) and place in the hot butter to sear. To get a nice sear, make sure the butter is quite hot and sizzles when you add the chops.
6. Sear the first side until browned (about 2 minutes). Do not move the chops while they are searing. Flip the chops and sear the other side for about 2 minutes.
7. Reduce heat to medium or medium low. Pour the reserved BBQ sauce around the pork chops and cover the pan. Cook over low heat for 3-5 minutes, or until internal temperature registers 135°F (57°C)
8. Remove from the skillet and let the chops rest for 5-10 minutes (they will continue to cook while resting).
9. Drizzle chops with the sauce and serve remaining sauce on the side.

Nutrition Notes (per chop): Calories 295; Protein 29g; Carbs 1g; Fat 18g; Sugar 1g

MODERATE — Makes 16 ribs from a 3-lb rack; 2-3 hours cooking time

Blueberry Glazed Baby Back Ribs

Great ribs shouldn't require a smoker, special rubs, or all-day babysitting. This foolproof method delivers tender fall-off-the-bone ribs using just your oven and a few hours of hands-off cooking time. The real game-changer is the blueberry balsamic BBQ sauce that brings sweet-tangy complexity without the artificial flavors and excessive sugar of store-bought sauces.

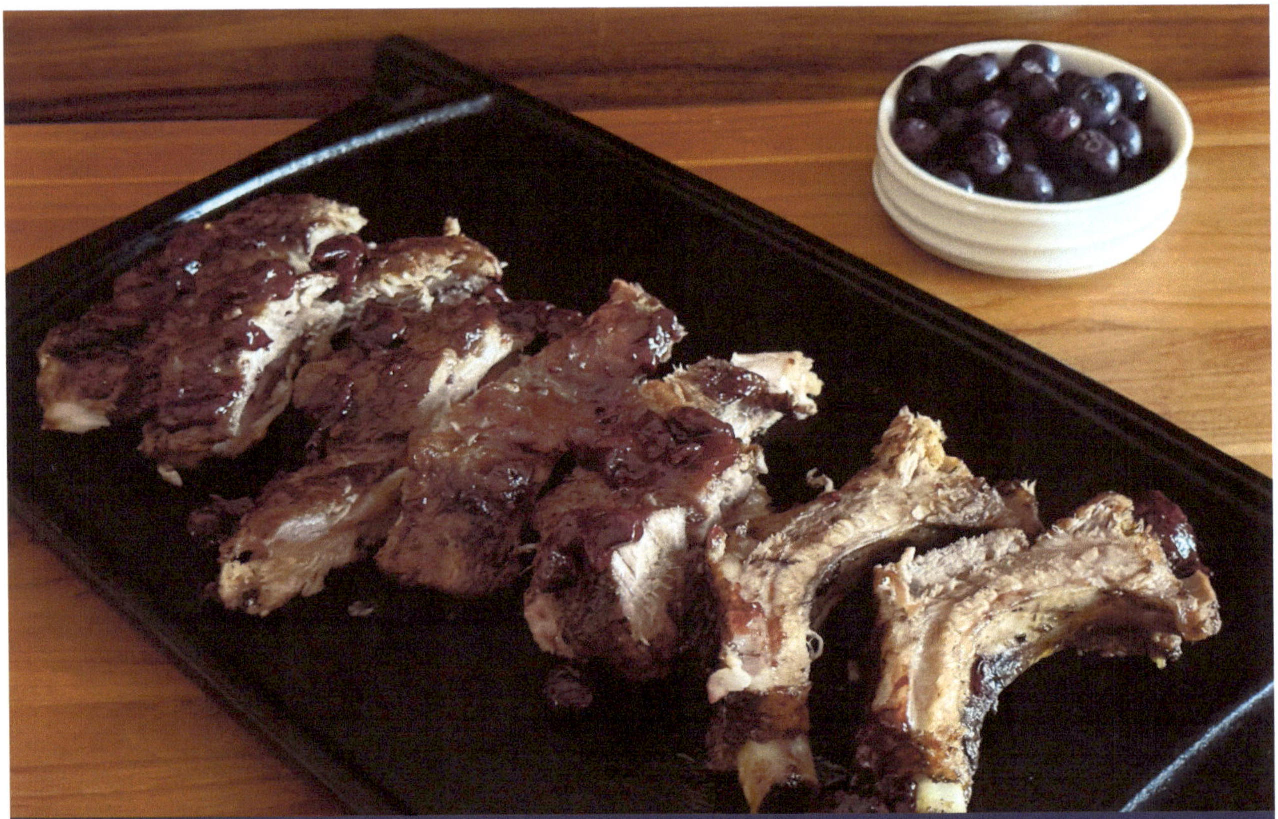

COOKING NOTES
- To remove the thin membrane, slide a knife under the membrane at one end of the rack and gently peel it away from the bones. It is helpful to grab it with a kitchen towel to pull it off instead of your fingers.
- Ribs can be stored in the fridge for about 4 days, or frozen for up to 3 months. Just wrap them very tightly.

INGREDIENTS

For the Ribs

3 lb rack of baby back ribs

2-3 tablespoons spice rub
(use your favorite or make my spice rub below)

For the DIY Spice Rub (optional):

2 teaspoons kosher salt

2 tablespoons paprika

1 teaspoon garlic powder

1 teaspoon onion powder

1 teaspoon cumin

2 teaspoons chili powder

½ teaspoon cayenne powder

1 teaspoon pepper

2 tablespoons brown sugar

1 teaspoon dry mustard

For the Blueberry BBQ Sauce:

½ teaspoon hot sauce (I use Cholula)

½ teaspoon liquid smoke

½ cup (3.5 oz) ketchup

¼ cup (60 ml) balsamic vinegar

3-4 tablespoons brown sugar (packed)

3 tablespoons Dijon mustard

⅛ teaspoon ground allspice

1 tablespoon oil

½ medium onion, chopped (75 g)

3 cloves garlic, minced

⅓ cup (80 ml) bourbon (optional)

3 cups (18 oz) blueberries
(fresh or frozen)

½ teaspoon kosher salt

DIRECTIONS

Make the Spice Rub:

In a bowl, whisk together all of the DIY spice rub ingredients. Alternatively use your preferred store-bought spice rub.

Make the Ribs:

Preheat the oven to 275°F (135°C).

1. Remove the thin membrane on the back of the ribs, as it can get tough when cooked (see the how-to in the notes below). Place the rack of ribs on a large sheet of foil on a baking sheet, meaty side up. If the whole rack doesn't fit on a baking sheet, cut it in half or to fit.

2. Season each rib generously with the DIY spice rub or the store-bought spice rub. Season front, back and sides of ribs. Wrap ribs tightly in the foil.

3. Bake ribs at 275°F (135°C) for 2-3 hours, or until tender.

Make the Blueberry BBQ Sauce:

1. In a bowl, mix together the first seven BBQ sauce ingredients (hot sauce through allspice). Set aside.

2. Heat 1 tablespoon of oil over medium-high in a large skillet, add chopped onions, and sauté for about 5 minutes until soft. Add garlic to the skillet and cook briefly (30 seconds).

3. Add bourbon (if using) and bring to a low boil for about 3 minutes. Add the blueberries and the reserved sauce mixture, stir, and return to a boil.

4. Add the salt, lower the heat and simmer for about 20 minutes, or until thickened to your preference.

5. **Finish the Ribs:** When ribs have finished cooking and before serving, unwrap the foil from the ribs, and turn the oven to broil. Brush ribs with the BBQ sauce. Broil for 2-3 minutes or until glazed.

Nutrition Notes (per 2 ribs): Calories 255; Protein 21g; Carbs 4g; Fat 18g; Sugar 3g

🥢🥢 MODERATE — Makes 2 game hens with enough sauce for 4 hens

Cornish Game Hens with Blueberry Cumberland Sauce

The challenge with impressive dinner party dishes is they usually require all-day prep and leave you exhausted before guests arrive. These glazed Cornish game hens look like you put in serious kitchen time, while actually being surprisingly simple. The secret is Cumberland sauce—a classic English sauce traditionally made with currant jelly. Since currant jelly is not readily available in typical American grocery stores, I have used blueberry jelly as a substitute. The Brits might call it heresy, but the flavor of this "Cumberland sauce" was truly remarkable!

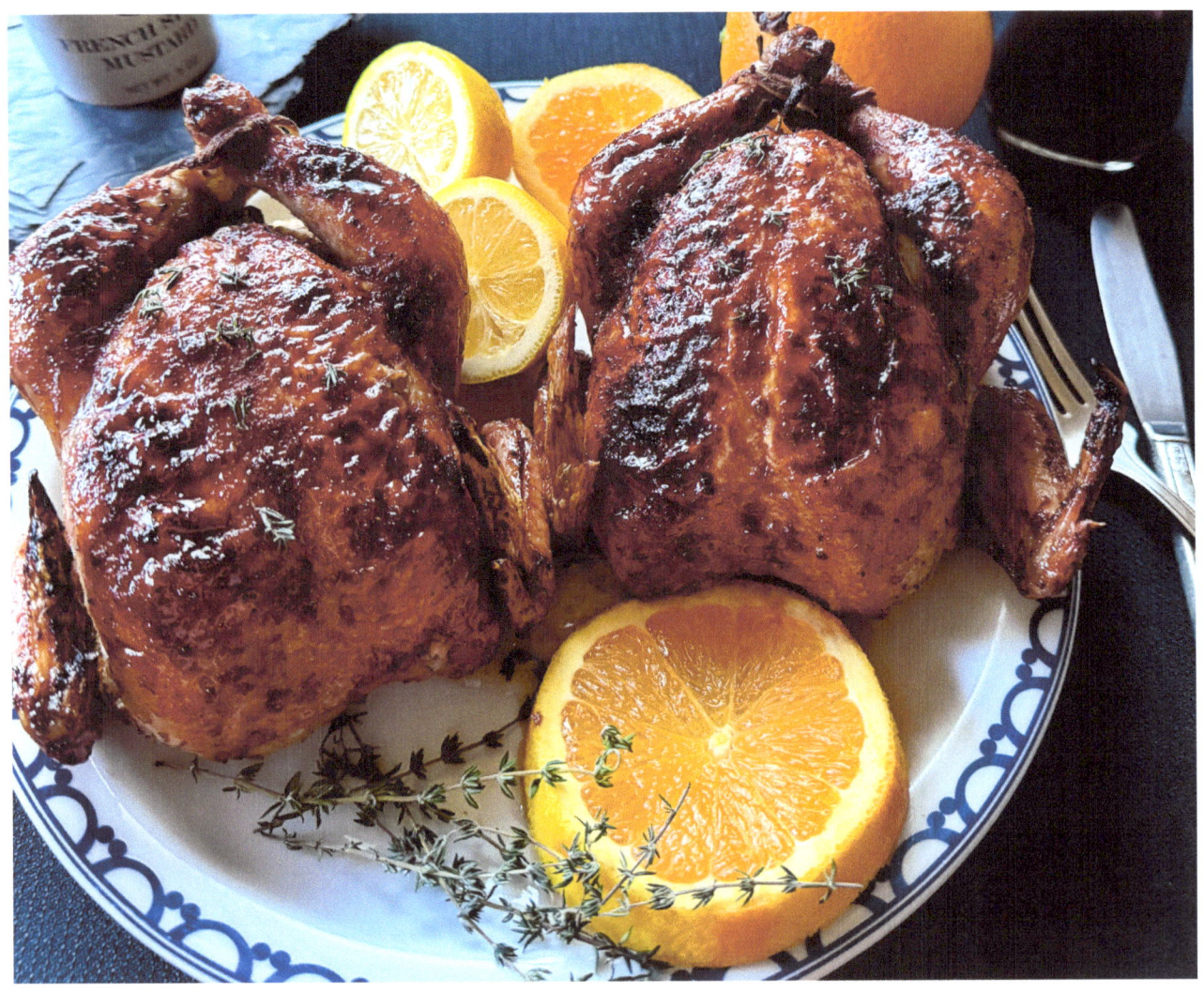

INGREDIENTS

- 2 (1-2 lb each) Cornish game hens
- 1-2 tablespoons unsalted butter
- 1 teaspoon kosher salt
- 3 lemons, divided
- 2 sprigs basil (~ 5-inches each)
- Handful of fresh thyme (about 12 sprigs)
- 2 tablespoons your favorite spice rub (I used paprika, onion and garlic)
- 1 cup (320 g) blueberry jelly
- 1 tablespoon orange zest
- 2 tablespoons orange juice
- 1 tablespoon lemon zest
- 1 tablespoon lemon juice
- ½ cup (120 ml) port wine (sweet port)
- 1 teaspoon Dijon mustard

DIRECTIONS

Preheat the oven to 400°F (204°C). Melt the butter for about 30 seconds in the microwave and then set aside.

Prep the Hens:

1. Pat the hens dry with paper towels, salt the inside cavity of each bird with ½ teaspoon salt. Slice one lemon and stuff the cavity of each hen with 2-3 lemon slices and a sprig of basil.
2. Slice another lemon and place thyme sprigs and 5-6 lemon slices in the bottom of a roasting pan. Place the hens on top of the herbs and lemons, and use a pastry brush to coat the hens with the melted butter. Sprinkle each with 1 tablespoon spice rub and about ½ to 1 teaspoon salt (omit salt if your rub has salt in it).
3. Roast in 400°F oven for 30-40 minutes, or until skin is turning brown and crispy.

Make the Sauce:

4. Zest one lemon and an orange, to get 1 tablespoon of zest from each. Cut the zested lemon and orange each in half and squeeze to get 2 tablespoons orange juice and 1 tablespoon lemon juice. Combine juices and set aside.
5. In a medium saucepan over medium heat, melt the jelly. Stir in the orange and lemon zest. Whisk the mustard and wine together in a small bowl and then add to the pan. Add the orange and lemon juices and simmer for 5-10 minutes, whisking occasionally. Taste and season with salt to your preference.

Glaze the Hens:

6. The skin should look deep brown and crispy by now (if not cook for another 5-10 minutes). Remove them from oven and use a pastry brush to coat them generously with the Cumberland sauce. Return to the oven for the last 15-20 minutes of cooking. A meat thermometer should register 160°F (71°C).
7. Remove and let them rest for 10 minutes. Brush with sauce once more and serve with remaining sauce on the side.

Nutrition Notes (for 1 hen and 2 tablespoons sauce): Calories 395 ; Protein 20g; Carbs 13g; Fat 27g; Sugar 9g

MODERATE — Makes 4 (¼-inch thick) burgers

Blueberry BBQ Bacon Cheeseburger

Gourmet cheeseburgers are the rage in summertime fare. The problem is they can get so fancy that they forget to actually taste good. This bacon-blueberry cheeseburger keeps everything down home and familiar, adding just a slight twist to surprise you with the unexpected. The sweet-tangy BBQ sauce doesn't compete with the bacon and cheese—it amplifies them, creating the kind of flavor combination that people will remember long after summer ends.

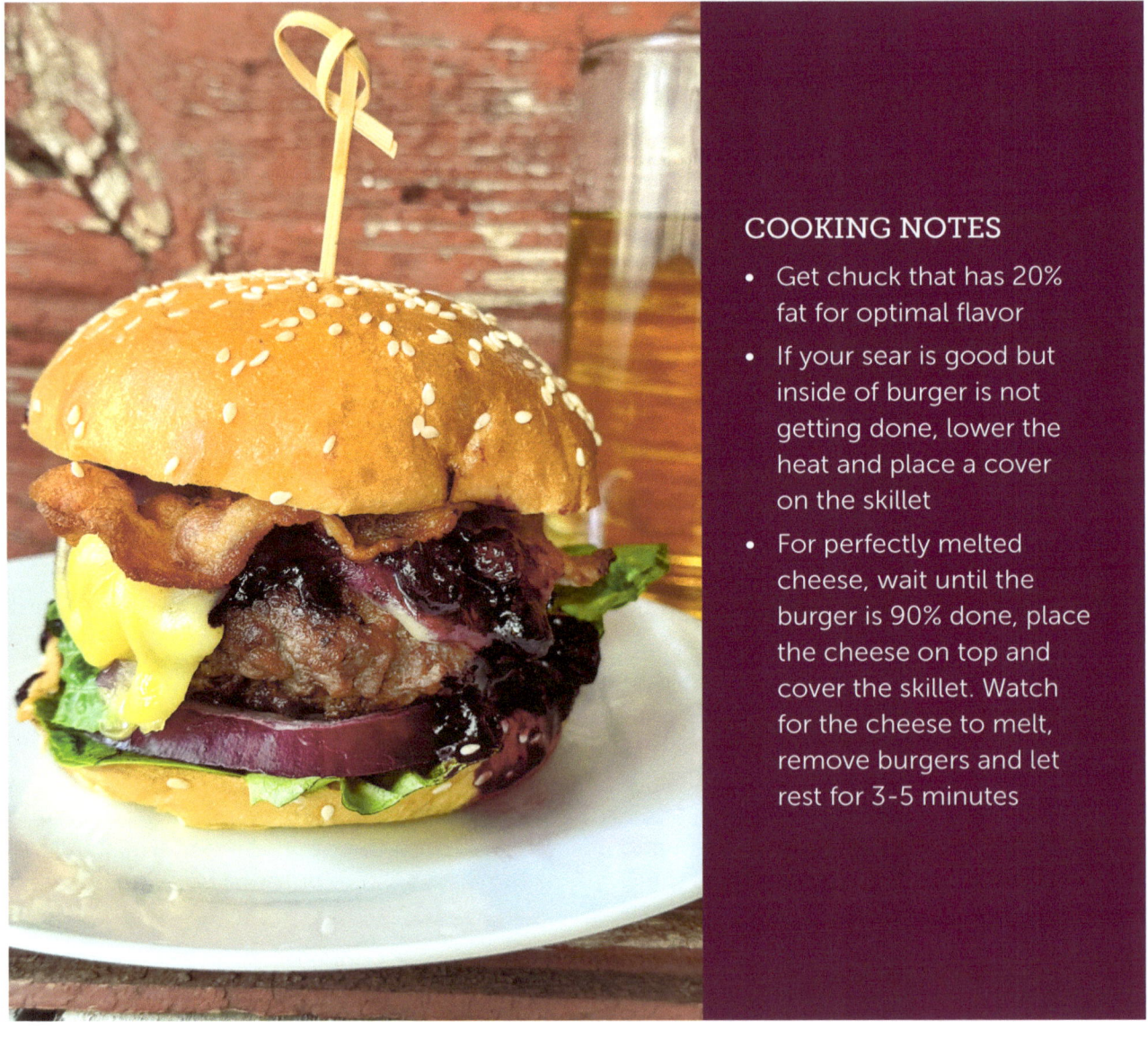

COOKING NOTES

- Get chuck that has 20% fat for optimal flavor
- If your sear is good but inside of burger is not getting done, lower the heat and place a cover on the skillet
- For perfectly melted cheese, wait until the burger is 90% done, place the cheese on top and cover the skillet. Watch for the cheese to melt, remove burgers and let rest for 3-5 minutes

INGREDIENTS

For the Blueberry BBQ Sauce:

½ teaspoon hot sauce (I use Cholula)

½ teaspoon liquid smoke

½ cup (3.5 oz) ketchup

¼ cup (60 ml) balsamic vinegar

3-4 tablespoons brown sugar (packed)

3 tablespoons Dijon mustard

⅛ teaspoon ground allspice

1 tablespoon oil

½ medium onion, chopped (75 g)

3 cloves garlic, minced

⅓ cup (80 ml) bourbon (optional)

3 cups (18 oz) blueberries (fresh or frozen)

½ teaspoon kosher salt

For the Burger:

5 oz (140 g) bacon strips (about 8 strips)

1 lb chuck ground beef (I like 80% beef/20% fat)

salt to taste

1 tablespoon refined olive oil

2 ½ oz (70 g) cheese (I use gouda)

4 hamburger buns

Optional additions:

sliced onions

lettuce, spicy arugal, or spinach

Mayonnaise, aioli, or tsatziki

DIRECTIONS

Make the Blueberry BBQ Sauce:

1. Stir together the first 7 ingredients (hot sauce through allspice).
2. Add 1 tablespoon oil to a large skillet and heat over medium heat. When hot add the chopped onions and sauté for about 3-5 minutes or until caramelized. Add the garlic and cook for 30 seconds.
3. Add the bourbon (if using) and bring to a low boil for about 2 minutes. Add the blueberries, the salt and the reserved sauce mixture, stir and bring to a low boil. Reduce the heat to low and simmer for about 20 minutes, or until thickened to your preference.
4. Cool and refrigerate until ready to use, up to 2 weeks.

For the Cheeseburgers:

1. Cut bacon strips in half crosswise and cook in a skillet over medium high heat until done to your preference (crispy or softer).
2. Form ground beef into patties about 4½ inches in diameter. Sprinkle with salt and use your thumb to add a small indent in the middle of the patty (helps to keep it from shrinking).
3. Heat oil in a large skillet until just starting to smoke and then add patties to the skillet (do not crowd).
4. Sear on one side about 4 minutes or until browned. Flip and cook on the other side about 3 minutes for medium rare. Add the cheese for the last 1-2 minutes and cover to melt the cheese.

Assemble the Burgers:

While the burgers are cooking, lay out your accompaniments and toast the buns. Layer the bottom bun with onion, lettuce, and mayonnaise, place the cheeseburger on top, drizzle with the blueberry BBQ sauce and top off with the bacon.
Get out the napkins and enjoy!

Nutrition Notes (per burger): Calories 634; Protein 32g; Carbs 24g; Fat 44g; Sugar 4g

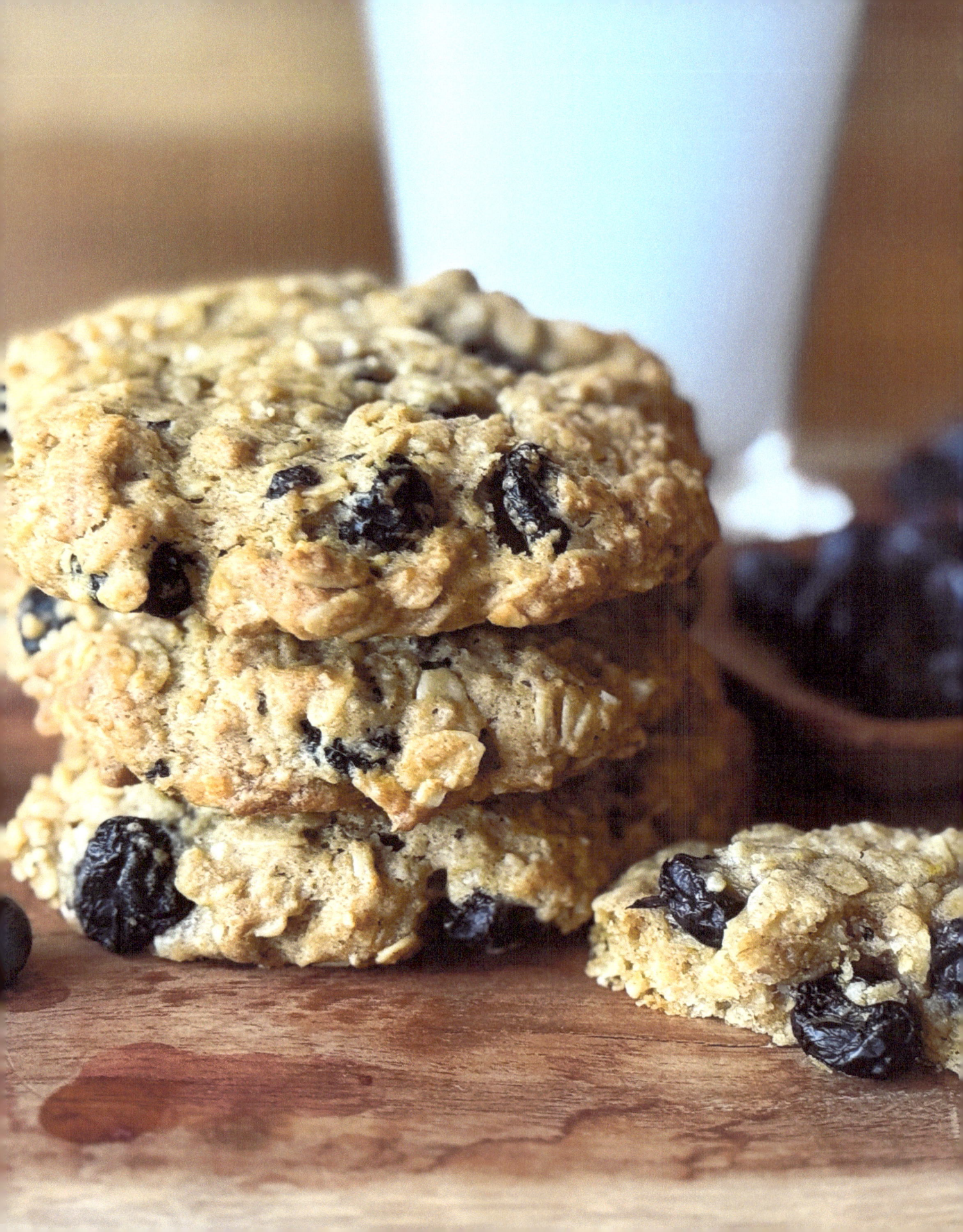

EASY RUSTIC DESSERTS

- 2-Ingredient Jam Tarts
- Crustless Blueberry Clafoutis
- Lemon Posset
- Skillet Blueberry Crumble
- Cornmeal Biscuit Blueberry Cobbler
- Cornbread Skillet Cake
- Blueberry Cornmeal Spoonbread
- Buckle Coffee Cake
- Oatmeal Cookies with Dried Blueberries
- Lemon Ricotta Blueberry Cookies
- Blueberry-Plum Galette

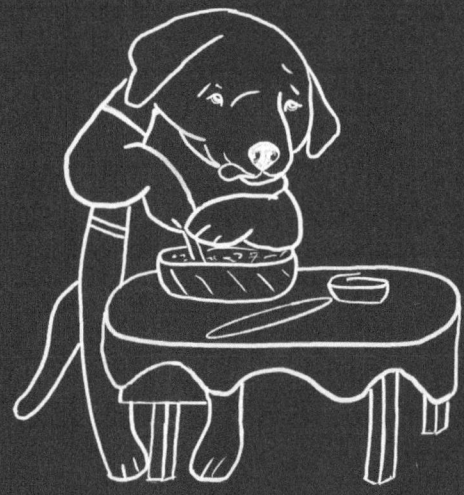

🥄 EASY — Makes 12 tarts (2 ½ inch diameter x 1-inch deep)

2-Ingredient Jam Tarts

These easy mini tarts made with a store-bought pastry dough and your favorite jams come together in 10 minutes! Jam tarts are a classic British treat, traditionally made with a "shortcrust dough". I wanted to make this recipe kid-friendly for the holidays, so I opted for a store-bought pastry dough. This makes it a 2-ingredient recipe that delights kids and adults alike.

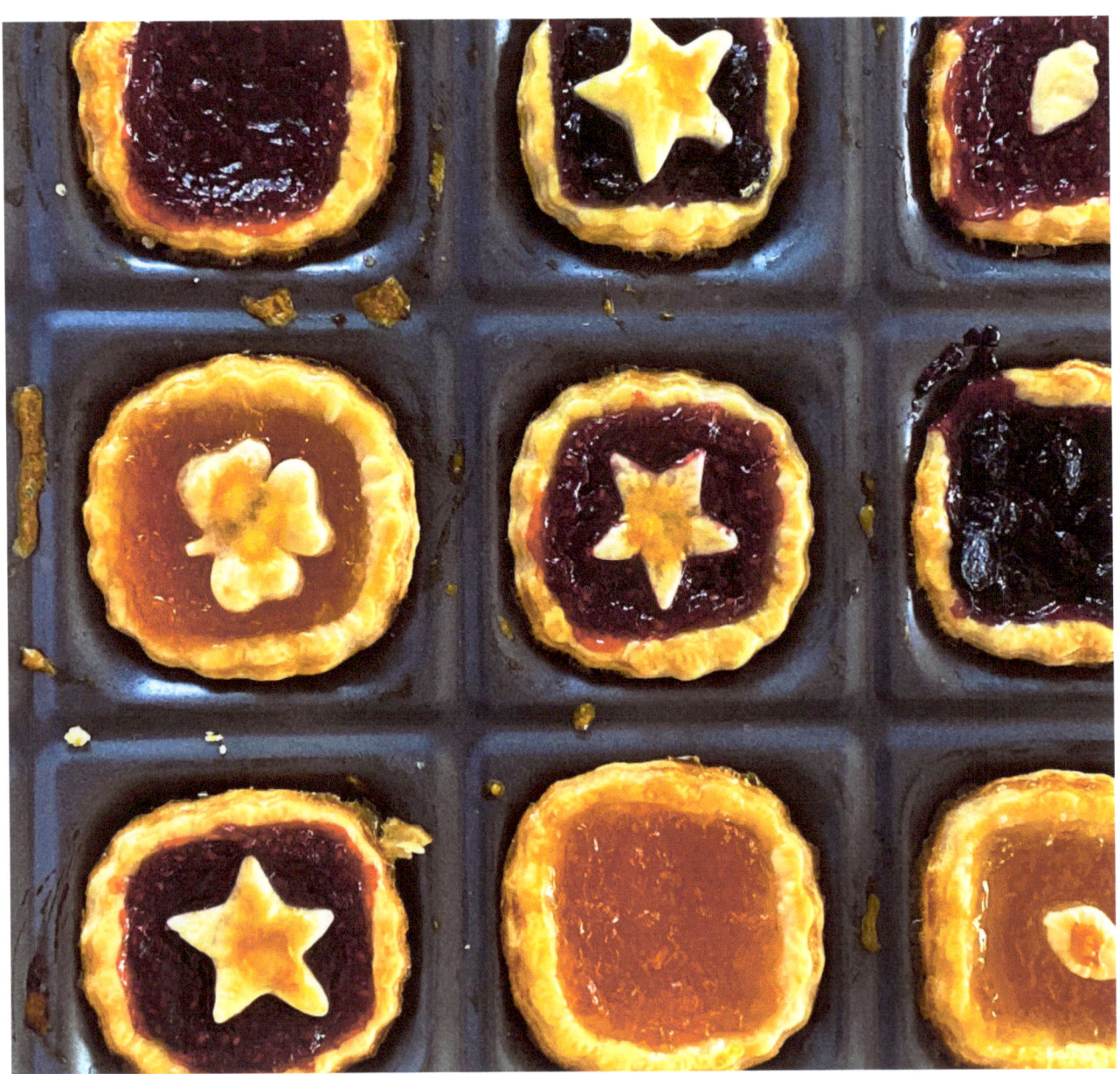

INGREDIENTS

½ package Pillsbury pie crust dough

12 tablespoons assorted jams

DIRECTIONS

1. Preheat oven to 375°F (190°C). Grease the tart pan with cooking spray or butter.
2. Unroll one of the pie crust rolls onto a lightly floured surface. Lightly flour a rolling pin and roll the pie dough out until it's 1-2 inches larger in diameter.
3. Use a round cookie cutter slightly larger than the individual molds in the tart pan and cut out 12 circles.
4. Gather the leftover dough and roll it out and use the small cookie cutters to cut out the shapes to place on top of the jam.
5. Use a thin spatula to lift the dough circles and place in the tart molds, gently pressing them into the molds.
6. Add about 1 tablespoon of jam to each tart. The amount of filling will depend on your mold, but try to fill each one about ¾ of the way to the top of the mold (too full and it will bubble over).
7. Gently press the small cutout shapes into the jam.
8. Bake for 15-20 minutes, or until dough is golden brown. If jam starts bubbling over, reduce temperature to 350°F (175°C). Remove when dough is golden brown. Cool thoroughly, the jam gets very hot!

COOKING NOTES

- The only modification I made to the ready-made pie crust dough was to roll it out thinner than it came in the package. The packaged roll was for a pie, and the tarts only have a tablespoon of jam in them, so you don't want the jam overwhelmed by a thick dough.
- The amount of jam to dough will vary based on your molds. Filling the tart mold ¾ of the way up to the top of the mold is a good estimate.
- Avoid overworking the dough, as it can cause shrinkage.
- Store any leftover dough, tightly covered in the freezer for up to 3 months.

SUBSTITUTIONS & ADDITIONS

- Substitutes for the jam fillings might include: Nutella, fresh fruit, pumpkin pie filling, savory ingredients that you might use in a meat pot pie.
- Substitute the store-bought pastry dough for shortcrust dough (Americans refer to this dough as shortbread dough).
- Do not use "puff" pastry dough, as it is too delicate for the jam fillings.
- Do not use phyllo dough, as it has no fat and won't have the same rich, airy quality of shortcrust pastry. My test recipes found that a refrigerated pie crust dough (I used Pillsbury) worked best.
- To make the dough turn golden brown, brush the crust with a beaten egg right before placing the tarts in the oven.

Nutrition Notes (per 2 ½ inch tart): Calories 24; Protein 1g; Carbs 8g; Fat 1g; Sugar 5g

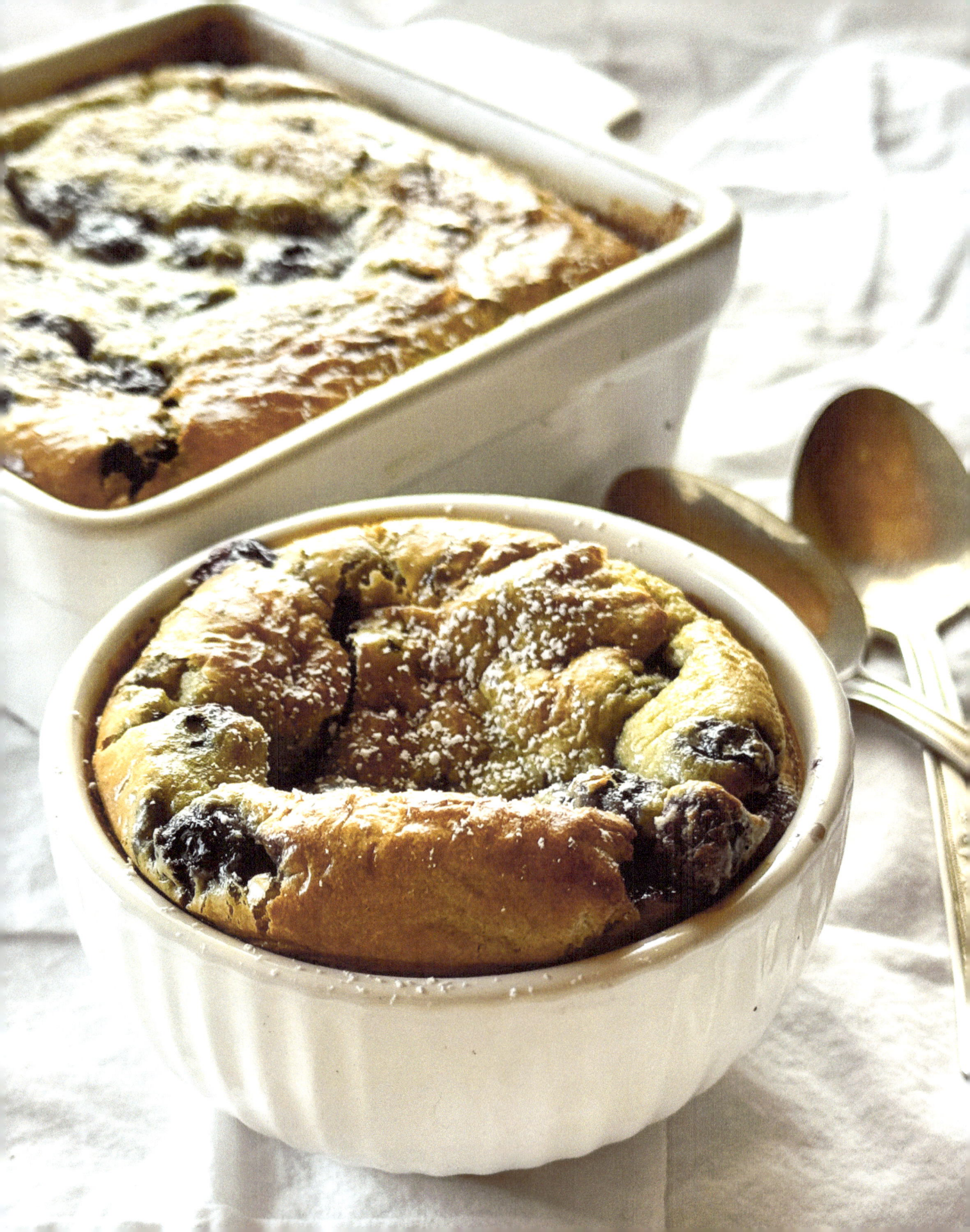

EASY — Makes 8 servings

Crustless Blueberry Clafoutis

I used to think French desserts were out of my league until I discovered clafoutis—basically a fancy name for "dump everything in a blender and bake." The problem most people have with elegant desserts is assuming they require pastry school skills, but this custardy tart proves that wrong. It literally took me 10-15 minutes to make. I made it crustless and low sugar to accommodate a low carb diet. You might want to add more sugar if you prefer desserts on the sweeter side.

INGREDIENTS

1 cup (120 g) almond flour

¾ cup (180 ml) almond milk

¼ cup (60 ml) heavy cream

4 eggs

¼ cup (50 g) granulated sugar

½ teaspoon kosher salt

1 tablespoon vanilla

1 teaspoon lemon zest

3 tablespoons (45 ml) Sambuca (optional)

1½ cups (9 oz) blueberries

SUBSTITUTIONS & ADDITIONS

- A classic clafoutis uses cherries instead of blueberries. When making this recipe with cherries, remove pits and cut them in half.
- Goat cheese would be a richer alternative to the almond milk and cream.
- Add more sugar if you prefer a sweeter dessert.
- Substitute Crème de Cassis (a black currant liqueur) for the Sambuca if you don't like anise flavor.

DIRECTIONS

1. Preheat oven to 350°F (177°C). Grease a 1 ½ quart baking dish (i.e., 9" round, 8 x 8 square, or 8 x 10 oval) with butter or cooking spray.
2. In a blender, add all the ingredients except the blueberries and blend to mix thoroughly.
3. Pour the mixture into the baking dish. Scatter the blueberries evenly over the surface. The blueberries may sink a bit but that is OK.
4. Place in the middle rack of the oven and bake 35-40 minutes or until golden brown on top.
5. Remove and let it cool in the baking dish. It will puff up while baking and deflate in the middle upon cooling. That is normal. It will still look and taste great.

COOKING NOTES

- Taste your blueberries before deciding on how much sugar to add. Some berries are quite tart and may need more sugar. Also, keep in mind that if you are using a liqueur, it will add some sweetness to the overall clafoutis.

Nutrition Notes (per serving): Calories 179; Protein 6g; Carbs 14g; Fat 12g; Sugar 10g

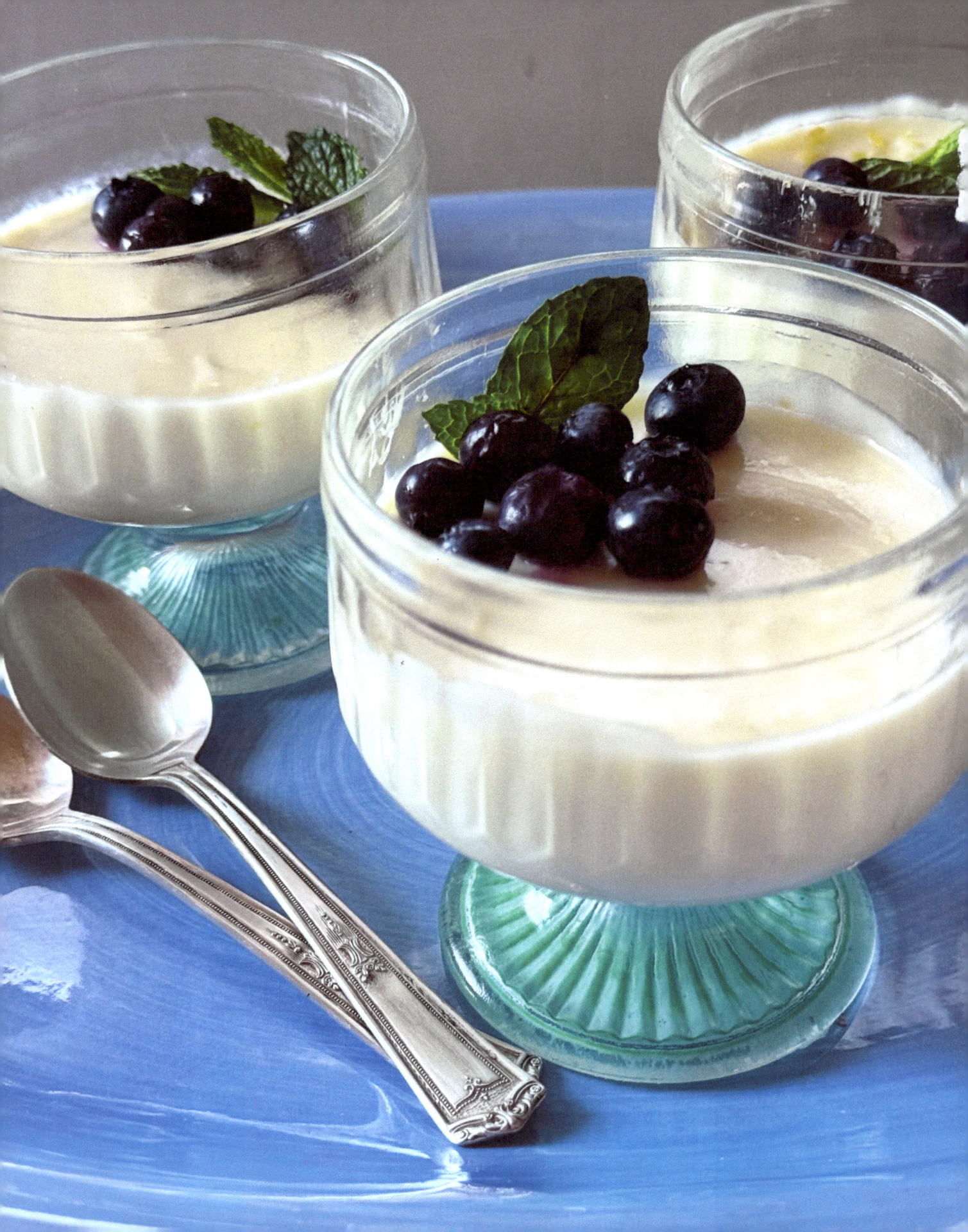

EASY — Makes 2 cups (4 servings)

Lemon Posset

Lemon and blueberries are a classic pairing, so I'm never without lemons when testing blueberry recipes in our commercial farm kitchen. The problem with most of the lemon-blueberry recipes was that the "lemon" flavor was subtle to non-existent. This simple lemon posset recipe finally delivered the lemon-forward tang I was pining for. The texture is silky-smooth and the tart flavor is balanced with a topping of of sweet blueberries.

INGREDIENTS

2-3 lemons

2 cups (473 ml) heavy whipping cream

⅔ cup (130 g) granulated sugar

1 teaspoon vanilla (optional)

⅓ cup (2 oz) blueberries

4 sprigs fresh mint for garnish (optional)

SUBSTITUTIONS & ADDITIONS

- Substitute oranges or limes for the lemons.
- Substitute strawberries or other small fruit for the blueberries

COOKING NOTES

- Make sure to use heavy whipping cream (fluid cream). Other forms of milk do not have enough fat and the custard will curdle when you add the lemon juice.

DIRECTIONS

1. Zest the lemons to get 2 tablespoons zest. Set aside 1 tablespoon zest for garnish and use the other 1 tablespoon for cooking in step 2. After the lemons are zested, cut them in half and squeeze the juice to get 7 tablespoons (75 ml) juice.

2. To a medium saucepan, add the cream, sugar, 1 tablespoon of the zest and the vanilla (if using). Bring to a low boil, stirring until sugar is dissolved. Reduce heat and simmer the mixture for 5-8 minutes, or until it is reduced to 2 cups. After 5 minutes, pour into a large glass measuring cup to check volume. If more than 2 cups, return to pot and simmer longer.

3. Remove from heat and pour into the glass measuring cup or a large bowl. Let it cool for 1-2 minutes.

4. Slowly stir in the lemon juice. Let it sit for 15-20 minutes.

5. Pour into your serving cups, cover with plastic wrap and refrigerate for 3 hours or up to overnight.

6. When ready to serve garnish with the reserved tablespoon of lemon zest, the blueberries and a little mint (optional).

Nutrition Notes (per serving): Calories 370; Protein 3 g; Carbs 29 g; Fat 29 g; Sugar 26 g

EASY — Makes a 9-10-inch diameter skillet (8 servings)

Skillet Blueberry Crumble

A "crumble" (aka "crisp") is the quintessential summer fruit dessert, partly because it is so delicious, but also because it is so easy and impossible to mess up. The classic crumble is essentially a layer of fruit covered with a topping of oats, flour, butter and sugar (and sometimes nuts), which is then baked in the oven and served with a generous dollop of ice cream. I keep a batch of the crumble topping in the freezer for any spontaneous cravings my family might have for this popular rustic dessert.

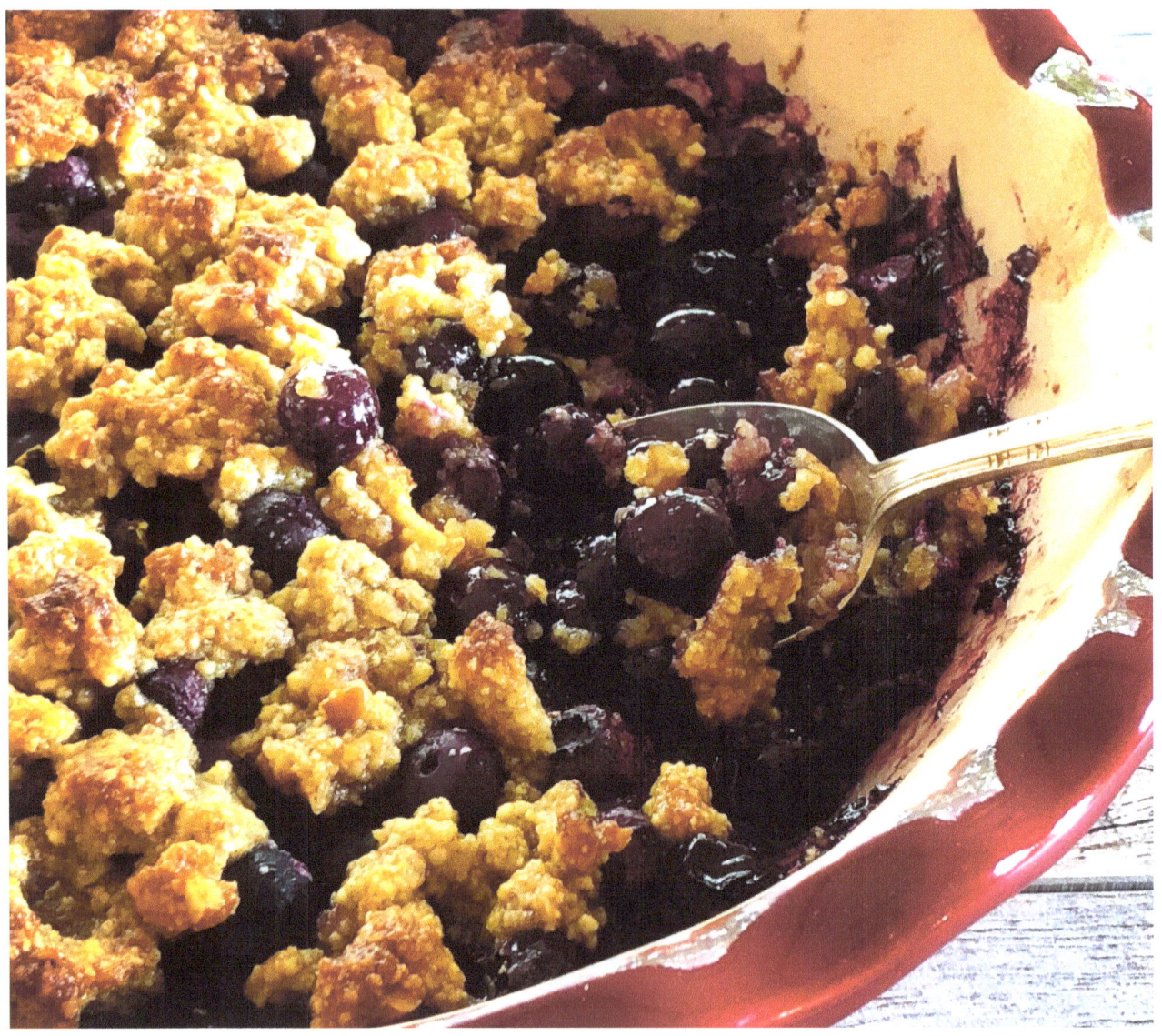

INGREDIENTS

For the Filling:

5 cups (30 oz) blueberries

½ cup water

¼ cup (55 g) brown sugar

1 tablespoon cornstarch

2 teaspoons lemon juice

½ teaspoon vanilla

For the Crumble Topping:

¾ cup (95 g) all-purpose flour

½ cup (100 g) brown sugar

¼ cup (23 g) rolled oats
(not quick oats or steel cut oats)

¼ cup (25 g) chopped nuts
(I use pecans)

Zest from ½ lemon

2 tablespoons granulated sugar

¾ teaspoon cinnamon

½ teaspoon ground nutmeg

¼ teaspoon kosher salt

½ cup (8 tablespoons/113 g) unsalted butter, cold

SUBSTITUTIONS & ADDITIONS

- Avoid instant oats as they will get mushy and avoid steel cut oats as they give a raw oat taste rather the crunchy sweet taste.
- Butter is the magic ingredient in a crumble topping. It offers texture and browning.

DIRECTIONS

1. Preheat oven to 375°F (190°C). Grease a 9-10-inch cast iron skillet or a 9-10-inch diameter baking dish with butter and set aside.
2. In a large bowl, combine all of the filling ingredients (blueberries through vanilla). Pour into your greased baking dish and set aside.
3. In another large bowl, mix together the flour, brown sugar, oats, nuts, lemon zest, granulated sugar, cinnamon, nutmeg and salt.
4. Cut the butter into small pieces and mix into the flour mixture with your hands or a pastry cutter or two forks until you have a coarse, pea-sized crumbs. It's OK if small pieces of the butter are not thoroughly incorporated.
5. Sprinkle the crumb mixture loosely over the top of the berries and place the skillet or baking dish in the oven. Bake, uncovered, until golden brown (35-40 minutes).
6. Let it sit about 10 minutes to consolidate the juices before cutting. Serve warm with ice cream or whipped cream.

COOKING NOTES

- Flour is my least favorite thickener, as you can taste it and it detracts from the flavor of the berries..
- If you want an even crisper topping, just add it for the last 15 minutes of baking instead of at the beginning.
- Storage: Store crumble topping in a sealed bag for 24 hours or freeze for up to 3 months.
- A 9" skillet with a depth of 2" is perfect for getting a bite of topping with each spoonful of fruit filling.

Nutrition Notes (per serving): Calories 340; Protein 3g; Carbs 52g; Fat 15g; Sugar 33g

MODERATE — Makes a 8-10 servings

Cornmeal Biscuit Blueberry Cobbler

Cobblers are distinguished from other old-fashioned fruit-dough desserts by the biscuit-style topping. It is called a cobbler because the top crust is not evenly spread over the filling like a pie crust, but rather "cobbled" and coarse (especially when the dough is dropped over the fruit by hand).

The biscuits for this cobbler are a light cream biscuit with a slight crunch from cornmeal. I've added my favorite spice of cardamom, which accents the vanilla and makes this cobbler a standout. Bonus is that it doesn't call for the buttermilk that cooks never seem to have on hand.

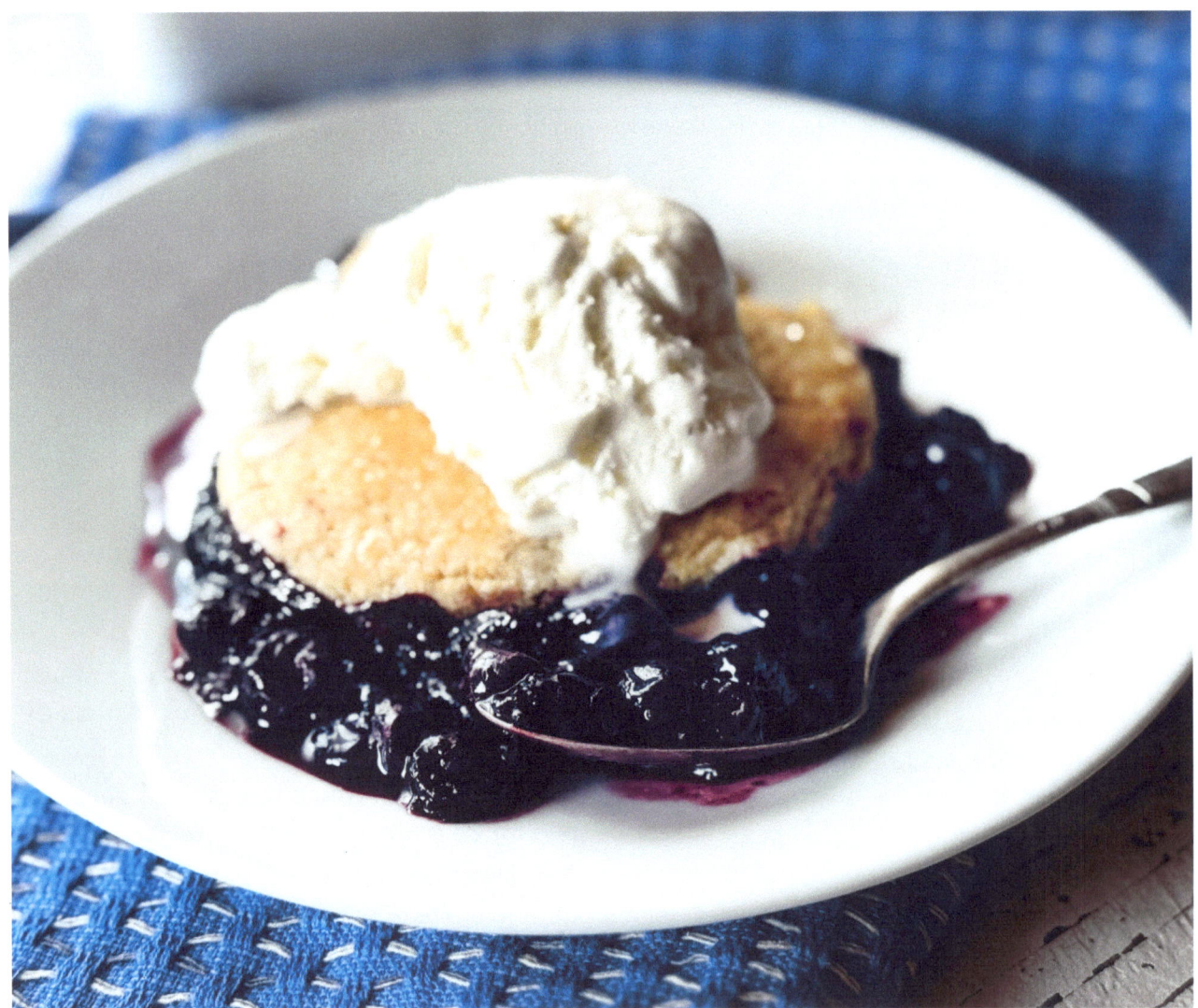

INGREDIENTS

For the Filling:

⅓ cup (65 g) granulated sugar

Zest and juice from ½ lemon

2 tablespoons instant tapioca

1 teaspoon ground cardamom

⅛ teaspoon kosher salt

4 ½ cups (27 ounces) blueberries

For the Biscuits:

1 ½ cups (180 g) all-purpose flour

¼ cup (30 g) fine-grained cornmeal

¼ cup (50 g) granulated sugar

2 tablespoons brown sugar

1 tablespoon baking powder

¼ teaspoon baking soda

½ teaspoon salt

½ cup (113 g) unsalted butter, cold

½ cup (120 ml) heavy cream

1 tablespoon cream or milk for biscuit wash (optional)

2 teaspoons sugar or turbinado sugar for topping (optional)

SUBSTITUTIONS & ADDITIONS

- If you have any fresh lemon verbena, chop up 3-4 leaves and add to the filling mixture.
- Another optional addition could be 2-4 teaspoons ground ginger.
- If you don't want to use heavy cream you can sub in ½ cup buttermilk or Greek plain yogurt with a little skim milk.

DIRECTIONS

1. Preheat the oven to 375°F (190°C). Butter or use cooking spray to grease a baking dish.

2. In a medium bowl, whisk together sugar, lemon zest and lemon juice, tapioca, cardamom, and salt. Fold in the blueberries stirring to coat with the dry ingredients. Pour filling mixture into the greased baking dish.

3. In a food processor, add flour, cornmeal, both sugars, baking powder, baking soda, and salt. Pulse a few times to combine.

4. Add butter to the processor, cutting it into small pieces. Pulse until butter and dough are the size of small peas. Add cream to the processor and pulse until dough is a coarse meal.

5. Lightly flour your countertop and use your hands to bring the dough together into a cohesive ball and place on the countertop. Flatten slightly and use a rolling pin (lightly floured) to roll it out to about ¾ inches thick. This will be an approximately 8 x 10 rectangle for 8-10 biscuits of 2 inches each (you may have some leftover dough). Use a round cookie cutter or the rim of a drinking glass to cut out biscuits (alternatively just use a large spoon or your hands for a more rustic looking cobbler).

6. Arrange biscuits on top of the blueberry filling, leaving spaces in between for berries to bubble up. Brush biscuits with a little milk or cream and sprinkle sugar over the top.

7. Bake for 40-50 minutes, or until biscuits are golden brown and berries are bubbling. Cool for 20 minutes before serving to allow fruit filling to set.

8. Serve with vanilla ice cream and enjoy!

Nutrition Notes (per serving): Calories 379; Protein 4 g; Carbs 52 g; Fat 18 g; Sugar 24 g

🥄 EASY — Makes a 9" skillet (~ 9 servings)

Cornbread Skillet Cake

Very easy and not too sweet, this cornmeal cake can be whipped up for an easy breakfast or drizzled with honey and enjoyed as a summer dessert. Making it in a skillet not only keeps the dishwashing to a minimum, but allows for golden brown, crispy edges. The result is more like a moist, tender blueberry cornbread than a traditional cake, and since it is designed around canned creamed corn and frozen blueberries, you can make it any time of year.

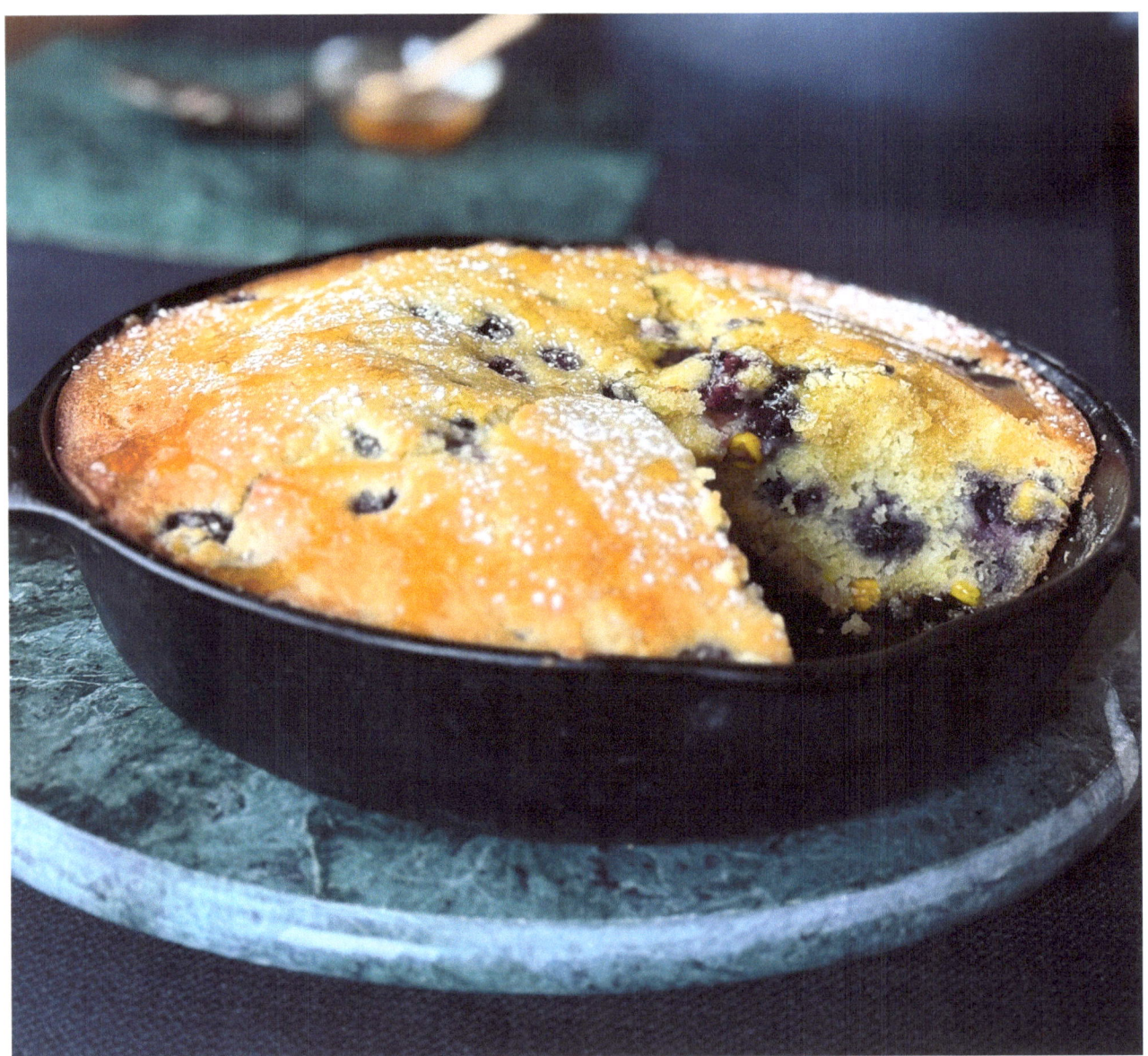

INGREDIENTS

½ cup (1 stick/113 g) butter, softened + 1 tablespoon for greasing the skillet

1 ½ cups (194 g) all-purpose flour

¾ cup (127 g) medium grind cornmeal

½ cup (107 g) sugar

1 tablespoon baking powder

¼ teaspoon salt

2 eggs, lightly beaten

1 14-oz can creamed corn

¾ cup (180 ml) whole milk

⅓ cup (80 ml) fresh lemon juice + 2 teaspoons zest

½ teaspoon vanilla

2 cups (12 oz) blueberries

DIRECTIONS

1. Preheat the oven to 375°F (190° C). Bring the butter to room temperature, or soften the butter in the microwave for 10-15 seconds, but don't melt.
2. Whisk together the dry ingredients (flour through salt) in a large bowl.
3. In a medium bowl, lightly beat the eggs with a wire whisk. Mix in the softened butter. Add the creamed corn, milk, lemon juice and zest, and vanilla and whisk all together until combined.
4. Add the wet ingredients to the dry ingredients and stir together until combined (do not overmix). Gently fold in the blueberries.
5. Grease the skillet with a tablespoon of butter and pour the batter into the skillet. Place the skillet in the oven and bake for 30-40 minutes or until the top is golden brown and a toothpick comes out clean when inserted in the middle.
6. Cool in the skillet for 10 minutes, and serve with honey drizzled on top.

SUBSTITUTIONS & ADDITIONS

- For extra crunch drizzle a coarse sugar (like turbinado sugar) on top of the cake before baking.
- Buttermilk can be substituted for the whole milk and will give the cornbread a more tangy flavor. Avoid lower fat or non-dairy milks because the cake won't taste as rich and moist.
- Substitute any of the small berries (blackberries, raspberries or strawberries) for the blueberries, or use a combination of berries.

COOKING NOTES

- If you want to use buttermilk for the tang and do not have any readily available, you can add 1 ½ teaspoons white vinegar or fresh lemon juice to ¾ cup 2% milk. Allow it to rest for 5 minutes before using.
- This can be frozen for up to 3 months. Bring to room temperature before serving.

Nutrition Notes (per serving): Calories 342; Protein 7 g; Carbs 52 g; Fat 13 g; Sugar 17 g

MODERATE — Makes 10-12 servings

Blueberry Cornmeal Spoonbread

Spoonbread is an old-fashioned southern dish that is something of a cross between a corn pudding, a cornbread, and a souffle. My mom, a quintessential southern belle from Louisiana, dearly loved her spoonbread (as well as her hush puppies and sweet potatoes). While I still hold the food memory of her spoonbread close, I've taken some liberties with her recipe and added blueberries and a sweet spice blend called Chinese five spice. She would not approve of the Chinese five spice, but I really like this spice blend with sweet baked goods.

COOKING NOTES

- The stiff peak stage of beating egg whites is when sharp tips form and stay standing when beaters are lifted. When whites are overbeaten, they look curdled and dry and you cannot fix them. Better to start over.

- Frozen berries often work better in baked goods as the color does not bleed so much. Don't thaw them, just use frozen but check the cooking time as they may take a tad bit longer than fresh.

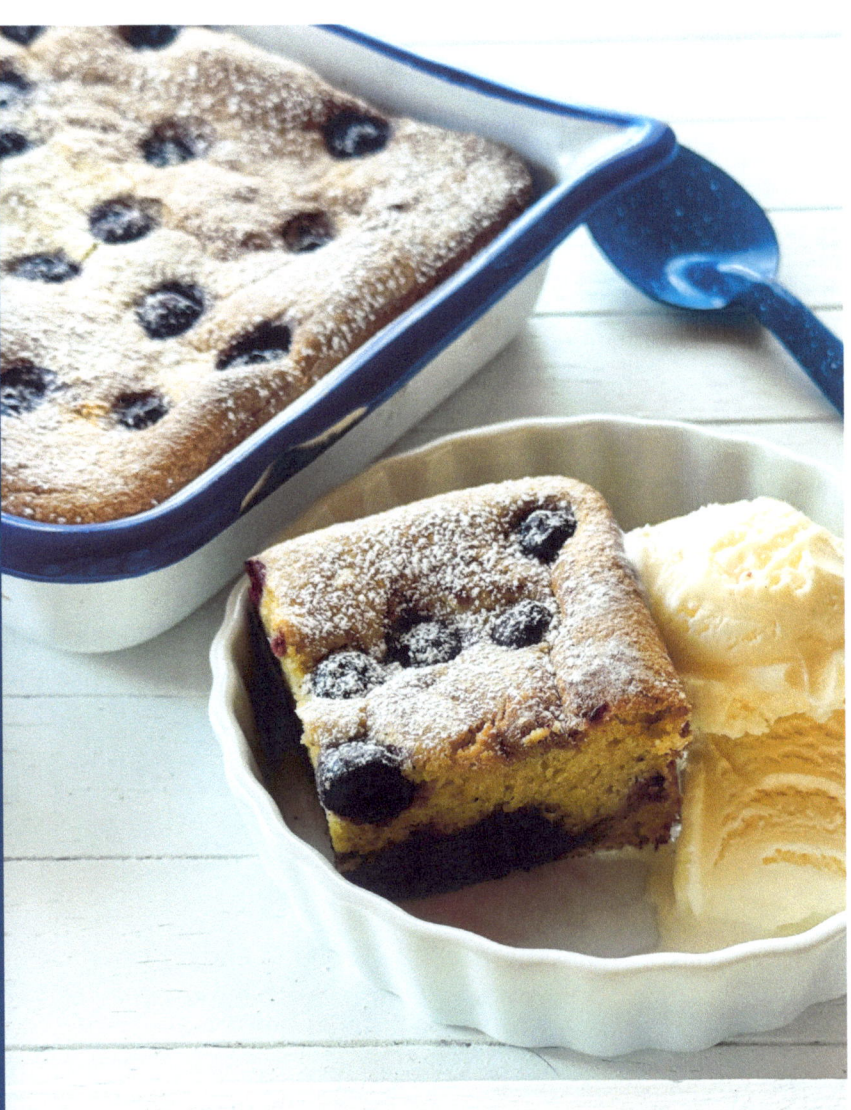

INGREDIENTS

4 eggs (separated into yolks and whites)

¼ cup (52 g) granulated sugar

1 ½ cup (360 ml) buttermilk

½ cup (80 g) brown sugar

1 cup (115 g) cornmeal (yellow or white)

2 tablespoons butter

1 teaspoon salt

1 teaspoon baking powder

½ teaspoon cinnamon

½ teaspoon Chinese five spice

1 teaspoon vanilla

1 tablespoon lemon zest

2 tablespoons heavy cream

2 cups (12 oz) blueberries (I used frozen)

DIRECTIONS

1. Preheat oven to 375°F (190°C). Grease a 2-quart or 8 x 8 baking dish with butter or cooking spray.
2. Separate the egg yolks from the whites into 2 separate bowls. Set the yolks aside for later use. In a stand mixer or hand mixer, beat egg whites with the granulated sugar until it forms glossy peaks. The peaks will have a point that stays upright. Keep them in the mixing bowl but set aside.
3. In a medium saucepan, heat buttermilk and brown sugar over medium-high heat until sugar dissolves and bubbles appear on the edges of the pan (buttermilk may get a little lumpy when heated, but that is OK). Slowly add the cornmeal, whisking it in thoroughly as you go. The mixture will become thick and mushy after a few minutes.
4. When the cornmeal mixture is a thick porridge-like texture, remove from heat and stir in the butter, salt, baking powder, spices and lemon zest.
5. Whisk the reserved egg yolks briefly and stir into the pan. Stir in the cream.
6. Check your reserved egg whites and make sure they are still fairly stiff (beat them a little more if they have softened too much). Gently fold the egg whites into the cornmeal mixture.
7. Reserve ½ cup of the blueberries for the top, and fold the other 1 ½ cups into the cornmeal batter.
8. Pour the batter into your baking dish and top with the reserved ½ cup of berries. Bake for 35-45 minutes or until the top is golden brown and a toothpick inserted into the center comes out clean.
9. Let it cool about 5 minutes before cutting to allow it to set.

SUBSTITUTIONS & ADDITIONS

- Substitute 1 ½ cups sour cream with ½ cup low fat milk (or water) for the buttermilk
- Substitute strawberries or corn kernels for the blueberries

Nutrition Notes (per serving): Calories 134; Protein 2 g; Carbs 22 g; Fat 4 g; Sugar 15 g

MODERATE — Serves 12: Made in a 8 x 8" baking dish

Buckle Coffee Cake

Growing up with a Southern mother born and bred in Louisiana, I had my share of those simple fruit and dough desserts with the funny names—buckles, grunts, pandowdys, sonkers or bettys. They all shared the same appeal: easy, inexpensive and fruit-forward. This blueberry buckle comes with a streusel topping which gives it a coffee cake feel, though it's also wonderful as a breakfast treat without the topping if you're short on time or want less sugar.

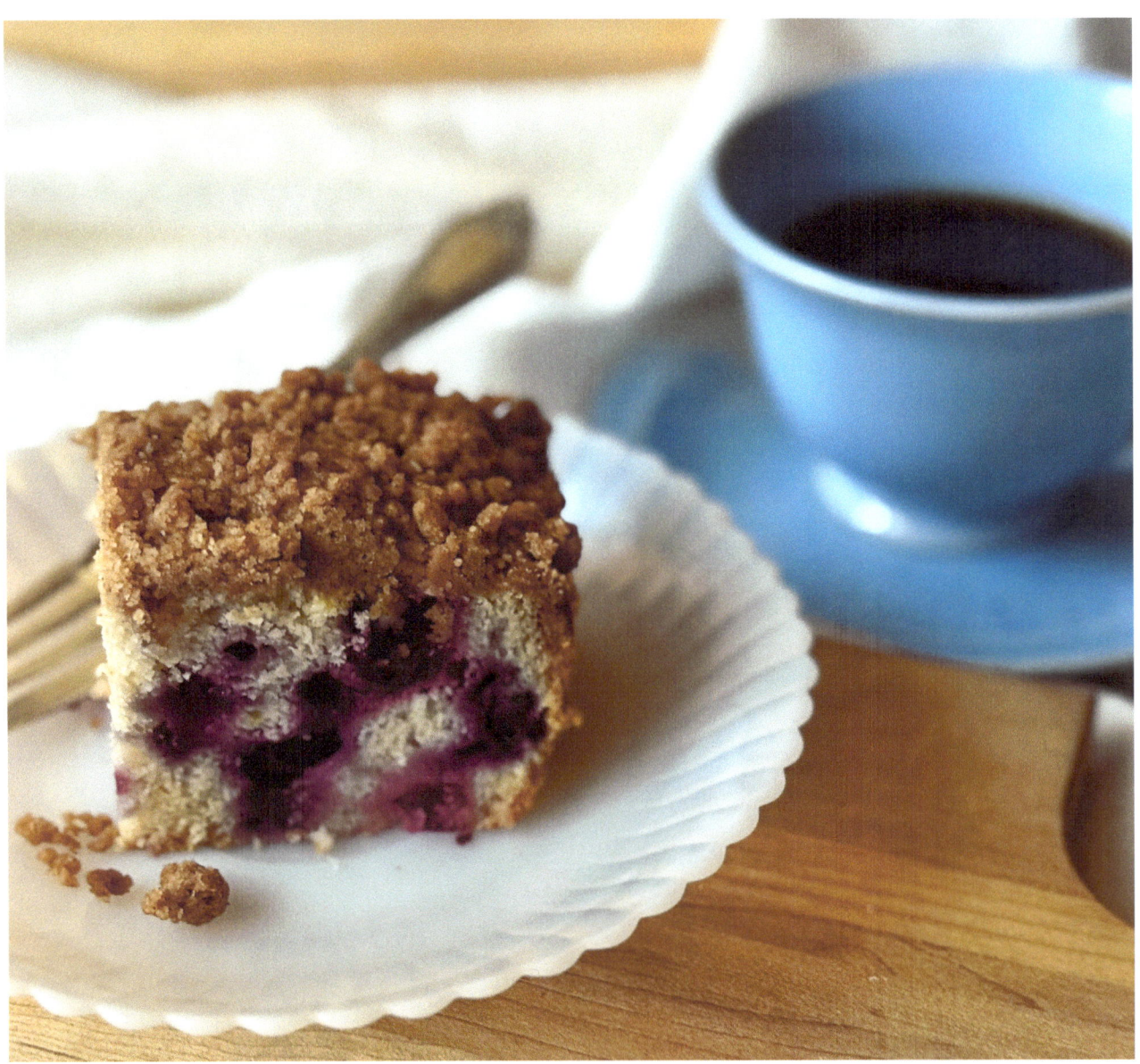

INGREDIENTS

For the Streusel Topping:

6 tablespoons (75 g) brown sugar

¾ cup (94 g) flour

2 teaspoons cinnamon

¼ teaspoon salt

5 tablespoons (75 g) unsalted butter, softened

For the Cake:

2 cups (240 g) all-purpose flour

2 teaspoons baking powder

½ teaspoon kosher salt

2 teaspoons lemon zest

½ cup (1 stick/113 g) unsalted butter, room temp.

½ cup (100 g) sugar

¼ cup (45 g) packed brown sugar

1 teaspoon vanilla

1 egg

½ cup (163 g) sour cream

2 cups (12 oz) blueberries (fresh or frozen)

SUBSTITUTIONS & ADDITIONS

- For a crunchier topping, add ¼ cup of pecans or almonds to the topping mixture.
- For a special treat, serve a square of buckle on top of a warm lemon sauce or lemon curd.
- Substitute ½ cup whole milk for the ½ cup sour cream for a lighter cake.

DIRECTIONS

1. Preheat oven to 350°F (177°C). Grease a 8 x 8" baking dish with butter or cooking spray.

For the Streusel:

2. In a bowl, stir together the brown sugar, flour, cinnamon, salt and softened butter until it resembles coarse crumbs. Set aside

For the Cake:

3. In a small bowl, stir together the first four ingredients for the cake (flour, baking powder, salt and zest). Set aside.

4. In a stand mixer with the paddle attachment (or using an electric beater), beat together the butter and the sugars until light-colored and creamy (not grainy), about 3-5 minutes. Then beat in the vanilla and the egg until just blended.

5. On low speed, beat in half of the flour mixture until just combined. Scrape the bowl and then beat in the sour cream until just combined (add a tablespoon of water if sour cream makes batter too thick for your preference). Beat in the remaining flour mixture until just barely combined.

6. Gently fold the berries into the cake batter (frozen berries are good here if you don't want the blueberries bleeding into the batter). Use a spatula and scrape batter into the prepared baking dish.

7. Scatter the crumb mixture evenly over the cake batter.

8. Bake 50-60 minutes, or until the topping is golden brown and a toothpick or knife inserted near the center comes out clean.

9. Let cool on a wire rack about 30 minutes before serving. Serve lukewarm with a hot cup of coffee or tea.

Nutrition Notes (per serving): Calories 302; Protein 4g; Carbs 45g; Fat 13g; Sugar 24g

MODERATE — Makes 2 dozen cookies

Oatmeal Cookies with Dried Blueberries

Although you can buy dried blueberries at the supermarket, they tend to be dried with a lot of preservatives to keep them pliable without molding. Using a dehydrator allows you to determine the texture—crisp and crunchy or raisin-like. This recipe trades the raisins for home-dried blueberries, resulting in a subtle fruity twist to the popular oatmeal raisin cookie.

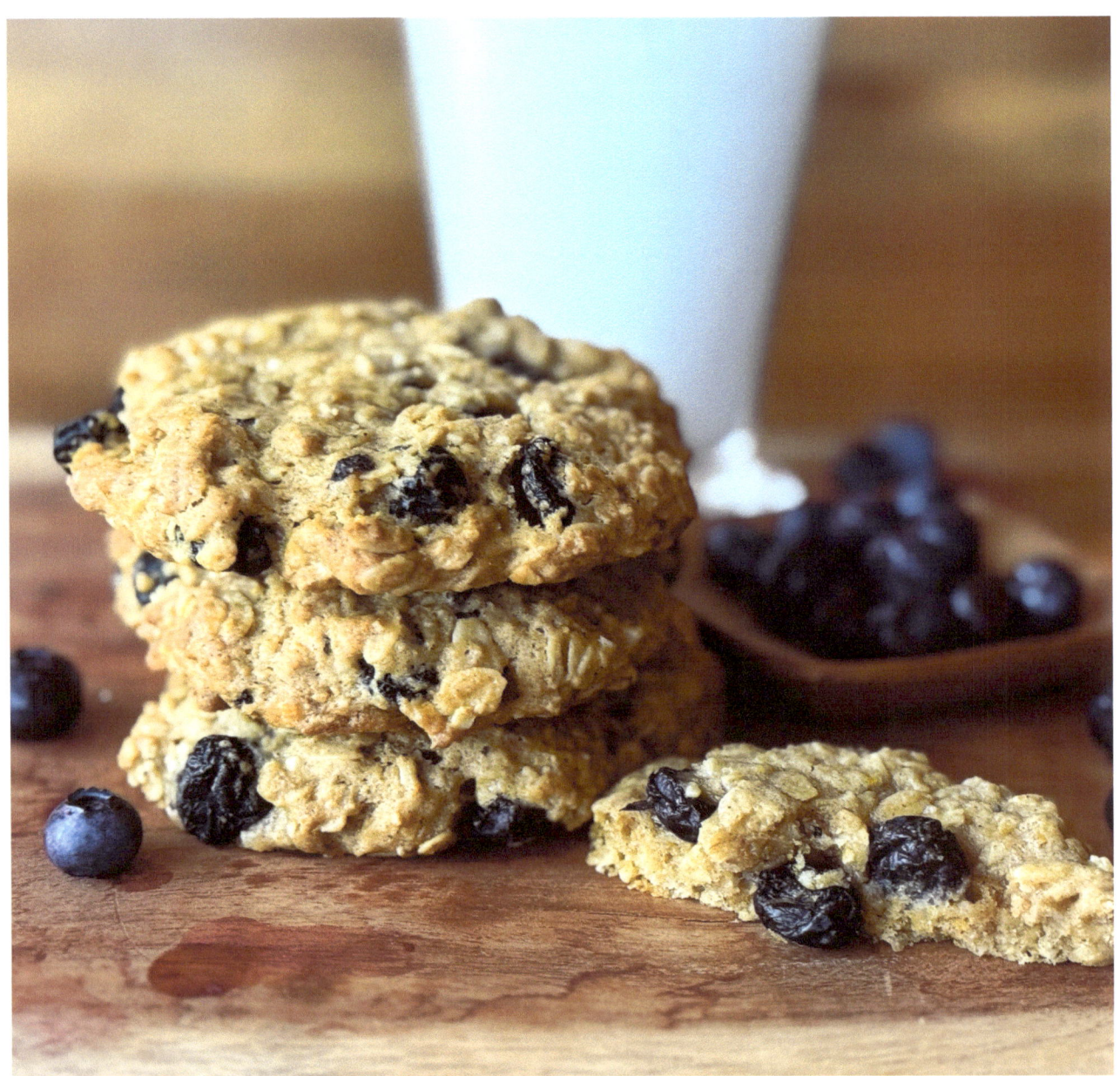

84 • THE BLUEBERRY COOKBOOK

INGREDIENTS

¾ cup (160 g) dried blueberries (see Foundational chapter for DIY dried blueberry recipe)

1 cup (226 g) unsalted butter, room temp.

¾ cup (135 g) packed brown sugar

¼ cup (50 g) granulated sugar

2 eggs, room temp.

2 teaspoons vanilla

1 ¾ cups (224 g) all-purpose flour

2¼ cups (202 g) Old Fashioned Rolled Oats

¼ teaspoon baking powder

1 teaspoon baking soda

½ teaspoon salt

2 teaspoons cinnamon

1 teaspoon lemon zest

DIRECTIONS

1. Soften the dried blueberries by letting them soak in a bowl of warm water for 15-30 minutes. Drain them thoroughly before adding to the batter.
2. Cream together the softened butter and the sugars in a stand mixer with the paddle attachment for 1-2 minutes, or until smooth (alternatively use a hand mixer). Avoid over-mixing or the increased air will cause cookies to go flat.
3. Add the eggs and vanilla to the mixer bowl and mix until well blended (1-2 minutes), scraping down the sides of the bowl as you go.
4. In a separate large bowl, whisk together the flour, oats, baking powder, baking soda, salt, cinnamon and lemon zest until thoroughly combined.
5. On low speed, slowly add flour-oat mixture to the wet ingredients in the mixing bowl, and beat until just combined. Drain the blueberries that have been soaking and fold the softened blueberries into the dough. The dough will be thick, but sticky. Chill the dough for 30-60 minutes in the refrigerator.
6. Preheat oven to 350°F (177°C). Remove the dough from the refrigerator and line two large baking sheets with parchment paper or silicone baking mats.
7. Gather about 2 tablespoons of dough into a ball and flatten slightly. Place each flattened ball 2 inches apart on the baking sheet.
8. Bake 12-14 minutes or until lightly browned. The centers will look under-baked but they will continue to set once removed from the oven. Cool on the baking sheet for 5 minutes. Remove to a wire rack to cool completely.
9. Cookies will stay fresh for about 1 week when covered. Alternatively you can freeze the dough for up to three months.

Nutrition Notes (per cookie): Calories 215; Protein 3g; Carbs 30g; Fat 10g; Sugar 13g

MODERATE — Makes 4 dozen cookies; Needs softened butter (2 hrs) & chilling time (1 hr)

Lemon Ricotta Cookies with Blueberry Buttercream Frosting

When most people think of Italian ricotta cookies, they picture something simple and understated. I've added a bit of flair to these beloved cookies by upping the lemon flavor and then topping them with a blueberry buttercream frosting.

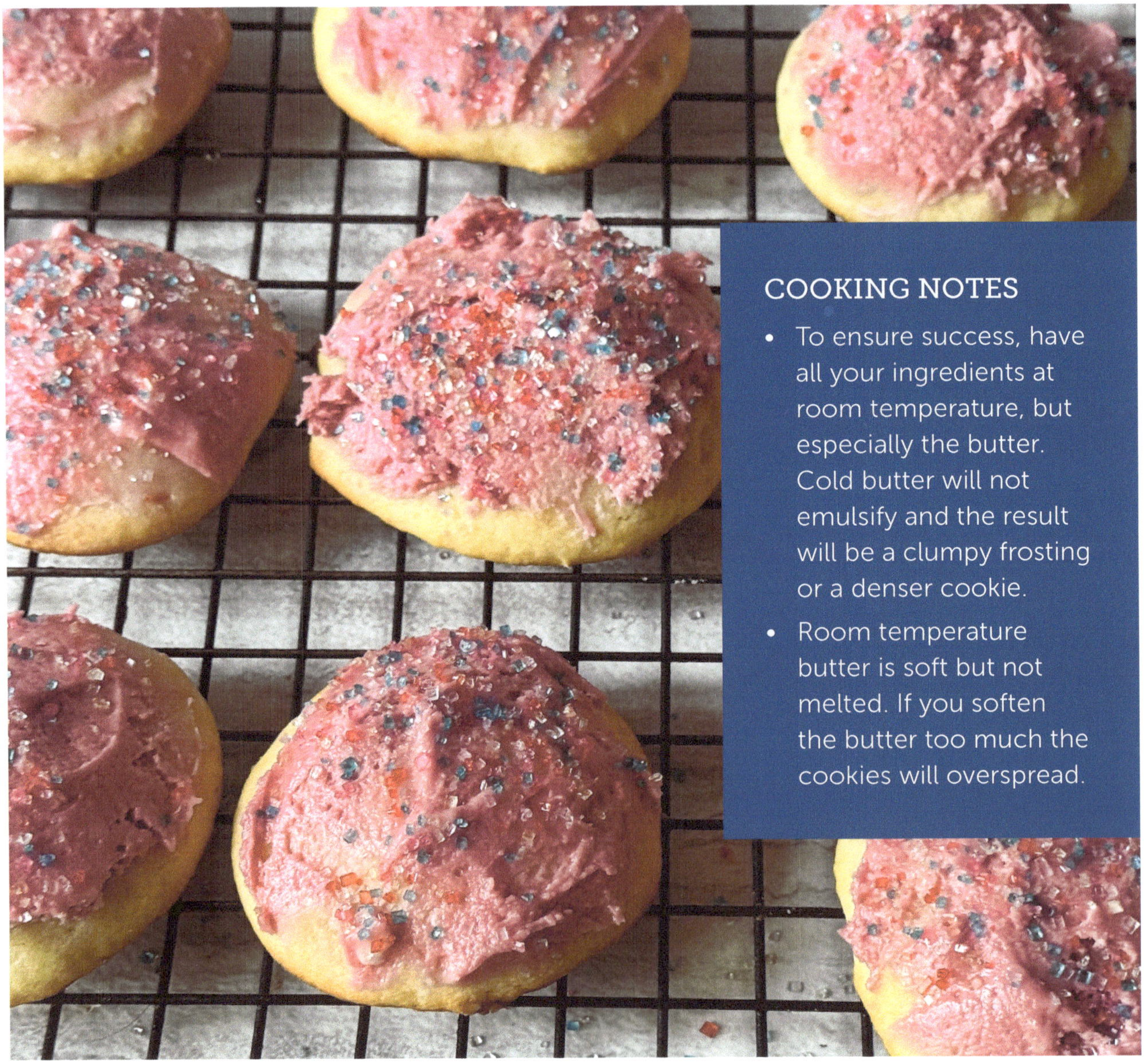

COOKING NOTES

- To ensure success, have all your ingredients at room temperature, but especially the butter. Cold butter will not emulsify and the result will be a clumpy frosting or a denser cookie.

- Room temperature butter is soft but not melted. If you soften the butter too much the cookies will overspread.

INGREDIENTS

For the Cookies:

2 ½ cups (313 g) all-purpose flour

2 teaspoons baking powder

½ teaspoon baking soda

¾ teaspoon salt

zest from 1 lemon

½ cup (113 g) unsalted butter, room temp.

1⅔ cups (335 g) sugar

2 large eggs, room temp.

15 oz (425 g) whole ricotta cheese, room temp.

3 tablespoons fresh lemon juice

2 teaspoons vanilla

For the Frosting:

¾ cup (170 g) unsalted butter, softened to room temp.

3 ½ - 4 cups powdered sugar

½ cup (130 g) blueberry jam or jelly

⅛ teaspoon salt

1 ½ teaspoons vanilla extract

2-3 tablespoons heavy cream (optional, if needed to thin frosting

DIRECTIONS

For the Cookie Dough:

1. In a large bowl, whisk together flour, baking powder, baking soda, salt, and lemon zest.

2. In a mixer, beat together the softened butter and the sugar for 1-2 minutes. On low speed, add the 2 eggs, softened ricotta, lemon juice and vanilla.

3. On low speed, beat in the flour mixture until just combined. Do not overmix. The batter will be sticky. Cover the bowl and chill in the refrigerator for 1 hour or up to 2 days.

For the Frosting:

4. In a mixer, beat the ¾ cup softened butter for 1 minute, or until creamy.

5. On low speed add the powdered sugar slowly so it doesn't fly out of the bowl. Beat in the jelly, salt and vanilla. If the frosting is too thick, add a little cream. If it is too thin, add more powdered sugar. Cover and refrigerate until ready to use.

Bake the Cookies:

6. When ready to bake, preheat the oven to 350°F (177°C) and line a couple of baking sheets with parchment paper or a silicone mat. Using a small ice cream scoop or a spoon, place rounded cookie dough balls on the sheet 3 inches apart (they will spread).

7. Bake 13-15 minutes, or until the edges start to brown and the center springs back when lightly touched. Allow cookies to cool for 30 min.

8. Use a small spatula to spread the frosting atop the cookies and add sprinkles if desired. Leftover frosting can be refrigerated for up to a week.

Nutrition Notes (for 1 cookie without frosting): Calories 82; Protein 2g; Carbs 10g; Fat 3g; Sugar 7g

Nutrition Notes (for 1 tablespoon frosting): Calories 44; Protein 0.04g; Carbs 5g; Fat 3g; Sugar 4g

🥄🥄 MODERATE — Makes one 12-14-inch galette (10 servings); Needs 1+ hour chilling time

Blueberry-Plum Galette

A galette (aka crostata) is a fancy name for a free form pastry. Galettes keep things simple—no crimping a pie crust or making a lattice. The whole purpose is to allow the fruit to be the star. A flaky buttery pie dough, a touch of natural sweetness from fresh fruit, and a dash of lemon zest are all that's needed for this easy rustic dessert.

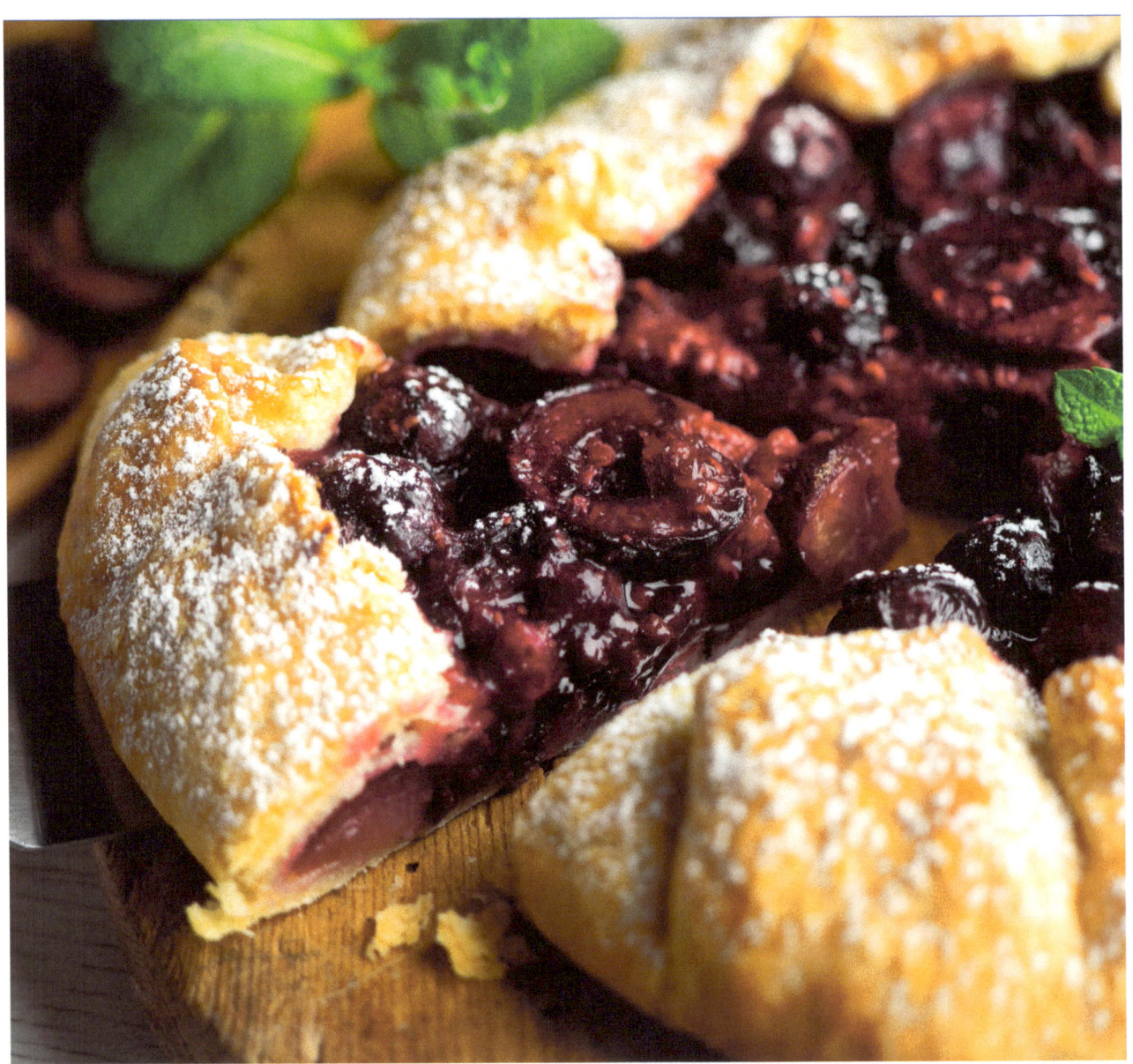

INGREDIENTS

For the Dough:

- 1 ¼ cups (156 g) all-purpose flour
- ¼ cup (30 g) fine cornmeal
- 1 tablespoon granulated sugar
- ½ teaspoon salt
- ½ cup (113 g) unsalted butter, chilled
- ¼ cup (60 ml) buttermilk, cold

For the Filling:

- 4 small plums, pitted and sliced
- 1–2 cups of blueberries
- 2–4 tablespoons granulated sugar
- 2 tablespoons cornstarch
- 1 tablespoon lemon juice
- ¼ teaspoon cinnamon or cardamom

DIRECTIONS

1. In a bowl, whisk together the flour, cornmeal, sugar and salt. Working quickly, cut the chilled butter into chunks and add to the bowl. Work in the butter until it looks like pea-sized crumbs.

2. Stir in the buttermilk. Using your hands, bring the dough together into a ball and flatten it into a 1-inch thick disc. Do not handle the dough too much or it will get warm and overdeveloped. Wrap the dough in plastic wrap and chill in the refrigerator for at least 1 hour or up to 3 days.

3. When ready to make the galette, preheat the oven to 425°F (218°C) and line a rimmed baking sheet with parchment paper or a silicone mat.

Make the Filling:

4. Toss all of the filling ingredients together in a large bowl, and allow it to sit for 10-15 minutes to draw out the fruit juices and activate the cornstarch.

Assemble the Gallette:

5. Remove dough from the refrigerator, and, on a lightly floured surface, roll it out to a 12-14-inch circle. This is a freeform tart, so don't worry about the shape. Transfer rolled-out dough to the lined baking sheet.

6. Spoon the filling into the center of the dough, leaving a 2-3 inch border. Fold the edges of the dough over the fruit, pleating as you go.

7. Brush the edges of the dough with an egg wash (1 egg and 1-2 tablespoons milk or cream whisked together), and sprinkle with coarse sugar.

8. Bake for 20-25 minutes, or until the crust is golden brown and the filling is bubbling. Cool for 10 minutes before serving.

COOKING NOTES

If you have not made a galette before and want more detailed instructions, see the recipe for galette dough in the Foundational chapter.

Nutrition Notes (per serving): Calories 198; Protein 3 g; Carbs 25g; Fat 10 g; Sugar 8 g

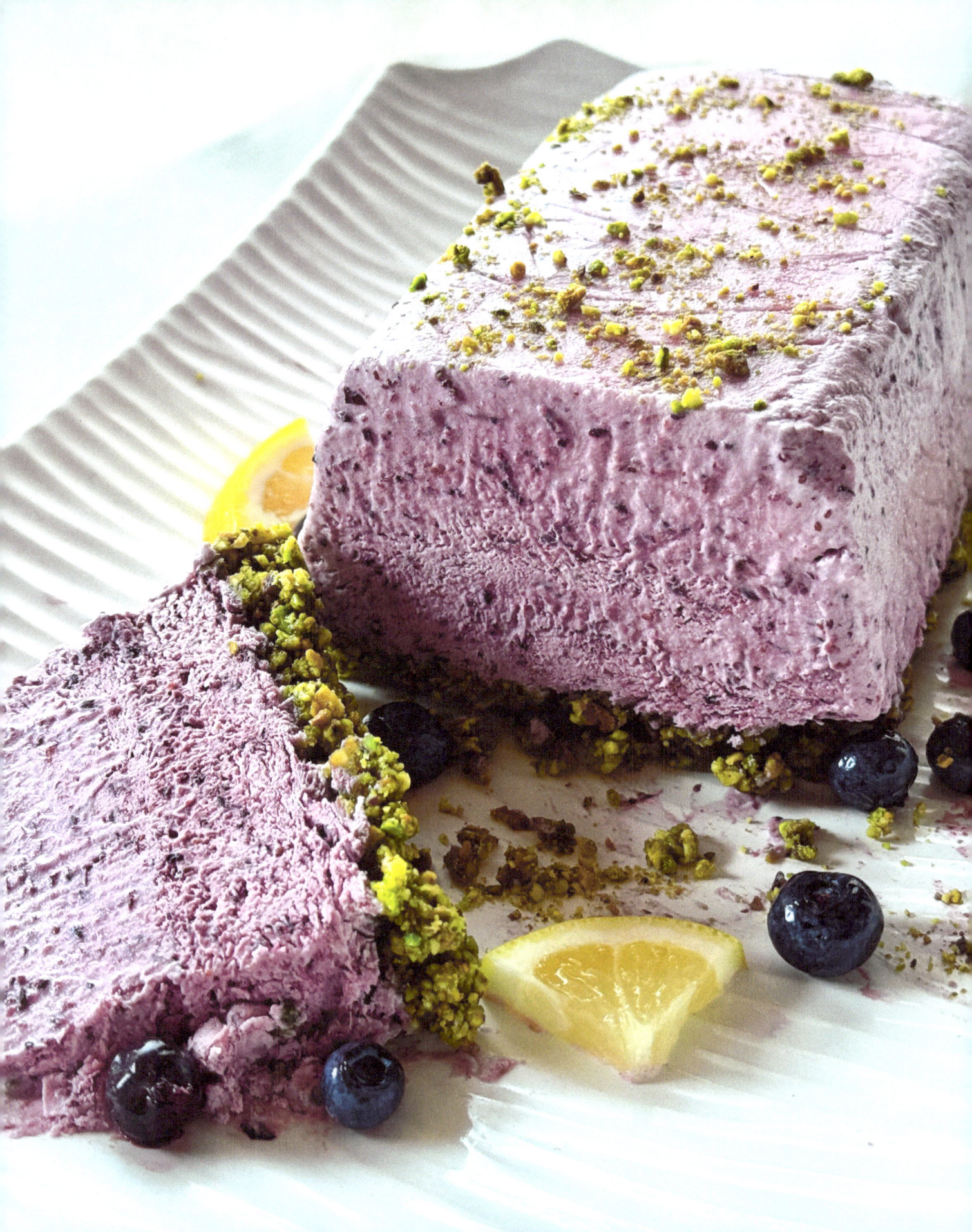

SUNDAY DESSERT PROJECTS

- No Churn Ice Cream Sandwiches
- Classic Blueberry Pie with Cornmeal Crust
- Finnish Blueberry Pie (Mustikkapriirakka)
- Chocolate Sheet Cake with Blueberry Cream Cheese Frosting
- Dutch Poffertjes
- Blackberry-Blueberry Poke Cake
- Lemon Blueberry Soufflé
- Semifreddo: No Eggs
- English Summer Pudding
- Poffertjes (Dutch Fair Food)

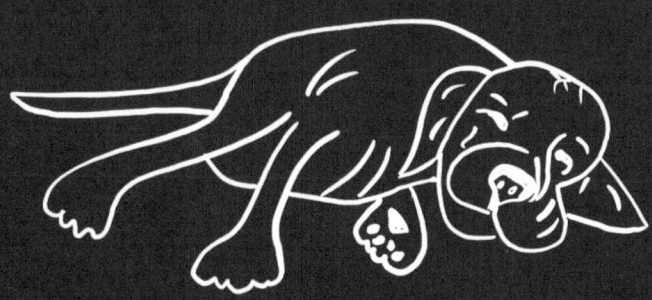

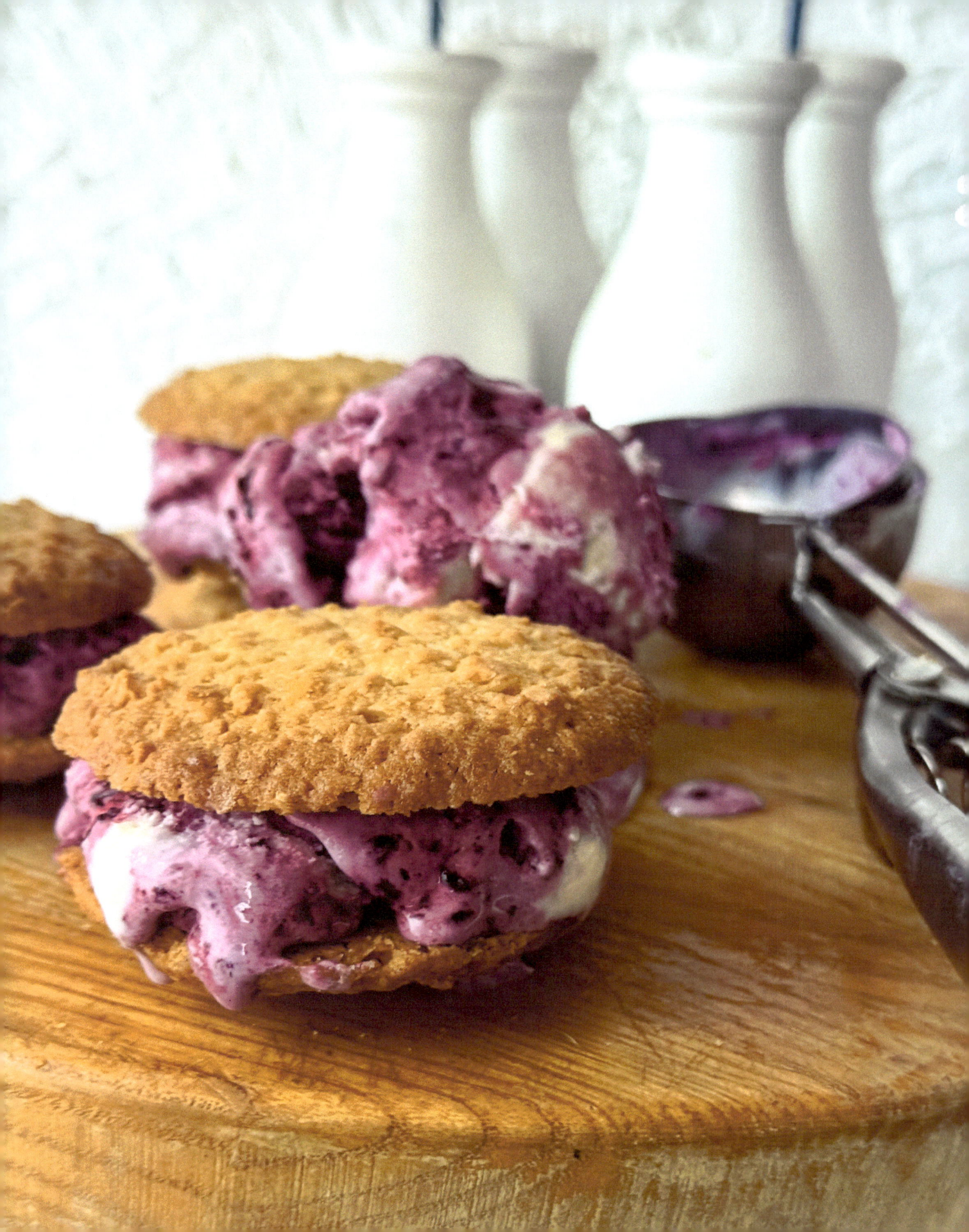

🥄 EASY — Makes 12; Requires 3+ hours chilling time

No-Churn Ice Cream Sandwiches

I have such strong memories of being a kid and living for those carefree hot summer days at the community pool (for me it was the Natatorium in Walla Walla, Washington). The day always ended with a soft, squishy ice cream sandwich from the concession stand. These aren't exact copycats, but they capture that same nostalgic feeling while actually tasting better than the originals. Store-bought cookies and ice cream infused with lemon and blueberries make everything easy– just mix, chill and assemble.

INGREDIENTS

1 tablespoon lemon zest

2 tablespoons lemon juice

1 cup (6 oz) blueberries

2 tablespoons sugar

1 teaspoon cornstarch

1 pint (16 oz) vanilla ice cream

24 cookies (use your favorite thin cookie; I used Tate's thin crispy coconut cookies from Costco)

COOKING NOTES

- If your compote is too thin, you can add another teaspoon of cornstarch or cook a little longer.
- If you don't like the texture of lemon zest in your ice cream, just add the juice and forgo the zest.

DIRECTIONS

1. Zest a large lemon and set aside 1 tablespoon of zest. Cut the lemon in half and juice it to get about 2 tablespoons of juice.

Make a Blueberry Compote:

2. In a small saucepan, combine lemon juice, blueberries, sugar, and cornstarch. Bring the mixture to a simmer over medium heat and simmer 2-3 minutes, mashing blueberries with a potato masher as it cooks. Remove from heat and let it cool.

Make the Ice Cream:

3. Remove the ice cream from freezer and let it sit on the counter to soften a bit while the compote cools. When ice cream is softened, stir in the reserved lemon zest. Swirl the compote into the lemon ice cream, without mixing it together thoroughly. You don't want a blue ice cream, but rather a swirl of blue and white ice cream. Cover the newly swirled ice cream and chill in the freezer for at least 3 hours.

Assemble:

4. Place a generous scoop of ice cream between 2 of your favorite store-bought cookies. Enjoy immediately. Alternatively, freeze the ice cream separately without the cookies so that the cookies stay crisp, and assemble when you are ready to eat.

Nutrition Notes (per sandwich): Calories 152; Protein 2g; Carbs 22g; Fat 6g; Sugar 15g

🥄🥄🥄 DIFFICULT — Makes 1 pie shell and lid (8-10 servings)
The dough needs chilling time (1 hour to overnight) + 15 minutes to warm up on the counter.

Classic Blueberry Pie with Cornmeal Crust

Although making pies can be a bit intimidating for the non-baker, if you're going to try your hand at it, this quintessential blueberry pie is a great place to start. I'll walk you through the steps, but even if your crust falls apart and the filling is too juicy, just top it off with ice cream and you'll still end up with something everyone will love. The cornmeal crust is extremely flaky and the blueberries are only slightly sweetened to allow the flavor to shine through.

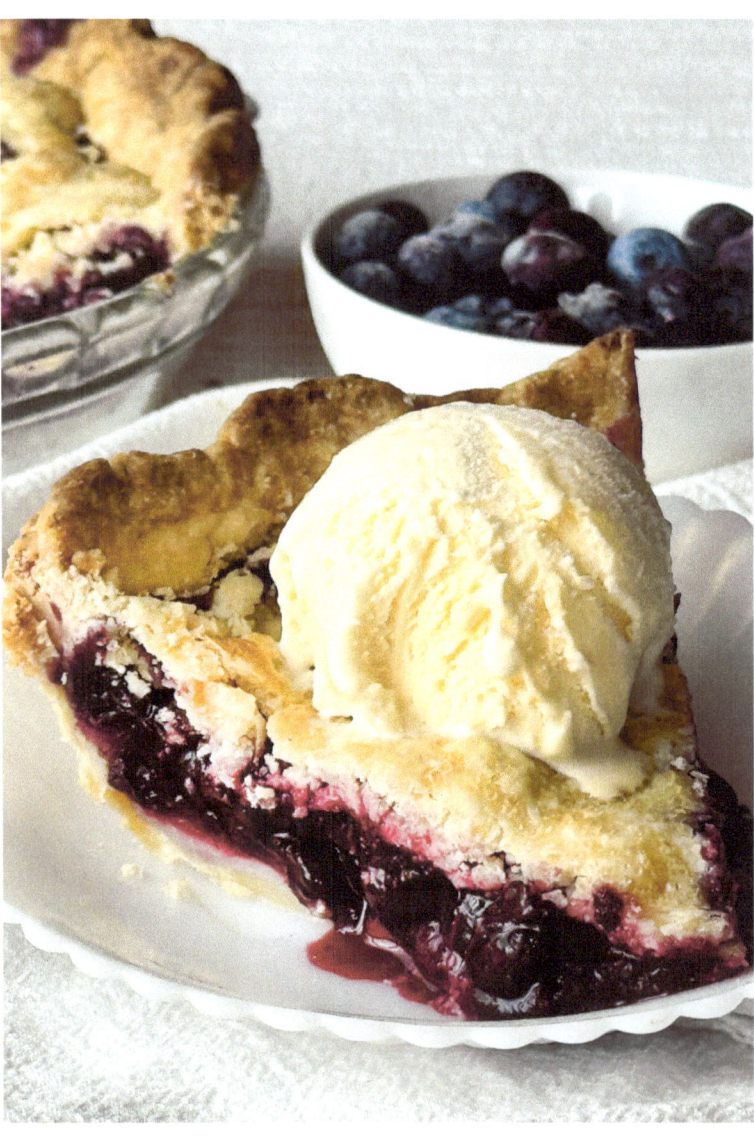

INGREDIENTS

For the Crust:

- 2 ½ cups (300 g) all-purpose flour
- ¼ cup (37 g) cornmeal
- 3 tablespoons sugar
- ½ teaspoon salt
- 12 tablespoons (168 g) unsalted butter, chilled
- ¼ cup (50 g) vegetable shortening (or lard), chilled
- 4 tablespoons (60 ml) ice water

For the Filling:

- 6 cups (36 oz) blueberries
- ¾ cup (145 g) sugar
- ¼ cup (30 g) flour
- 2 tablespoons cornstarch
- 2 tablespoons lemon juice
- 1 teaspoon lemon zest
- ½ teaspoon ginger
- ⅛ teaspoon salt

DIRECTIONS

For the Crust:

1. Fill a small bowl with ice water. In a food processor pulse together the flour, cornmeal, sugar and salt until combined. Cut the butter and shortening into chunks over the processor bowl and pulse until you get a coarse meal texture. Add the ice water and pulse just enough to bring the dough together.

2. Empty the dough onto the counter and form into a ball (dough will be thick). Divide the dough into two even balls and flatten each into a disc. Do not knead the dough—work it as little as possible. Wrap each disc in plastic wrap and chill for at least 1 hour or up to 1 day ahead.

For the Filling:

3. Combine blueberries, sugar, flour, cornstarch, lemon juice, lemon zest, ginger and salt in a large bowl and toss all ingredients together with a spoon or your hands. Set aside for 30 minutes (can be kept covered in the refrigerator for 24 hours).

4. Assemble the pie: When ready to make the pie, remove the dough and filling from the refrigerator and let them sit for about 10-15 minutes to reach room temperature. While the dough is warming up, preheat the oven to 400°F (204°C) and grease your pie plate with butter or cooking spray.

5. Place the first dough disc between 2 pieces of parchment paper and roll out to a 12-inch round. Peel off the top piece of parchment paper and invert the dough round onto the pie plate, leaving a generous overhang. Peel off the top parchment paper and gently press the dough into the plate (if it cracks, just wet your fingers and smooth it back together). Add the blueberry filling to the pie.

6. Repeat the rollout process with the second dough disc and place it over the top of the filling, centering as much as possible. Peel off the top piece of parchment paper and crimp the dough together around the perimeter of the pie. You can get fancy and flute the edges or just push the top dough together with the bottom overhang to form a simple crust. Use a sharp knife and make five 2-3" slits on the top.

7. Brush the middle of the dough (not the edges) with a little milk or cream and sprinkle with sugar (turbinado sugar if you have it). This will help mask any small cracks in the top crust and make the crust a visually appealing golden brown with sparkles.

8. Bake for 15 minutes and then reduce heat to 350°F (177°C) without opening the oven door. Continue baking for about 1 hour and 15 minutes, or until the crust is golden brown and the filling is bubbling through the slits in the crust. Look for the bubbling juices so you don't underbake the pie, or it will be soupy.

9. If the crust along the rim starts to get too dark you can cover it with a little aluminum foil.

10. Cool on a rack for at least 4 hours for the filling to set. Don't cut into it while it is still warm or it will be too juicy. Serve with ice cream! The pie can be refrigerated, covered, for up to 5 days.

Nutrition Notes (for 10 servings): 437 Calories; Protein 4g; Carbs 58g; Fat 22g; Sugar 28g

MODERATE – Makes a 10" tart (about 10 slices)

Finnish Blueberry Pie (Mustikkapriirakka)

OMG, this Nordic pie is so good I ate half of it as soon as I took the photo. It differs from a standard American blueberry pie in that you don't roll out the crust (none of that "crimping") and the filling is basically a sour cream custard poured into a pie crust which has been massaged into a tart pan or a pie pan and then packed with fresh or frozen blueberries. The result is something between a pie, a tart and a cheesecake that's absolutely irresistible.

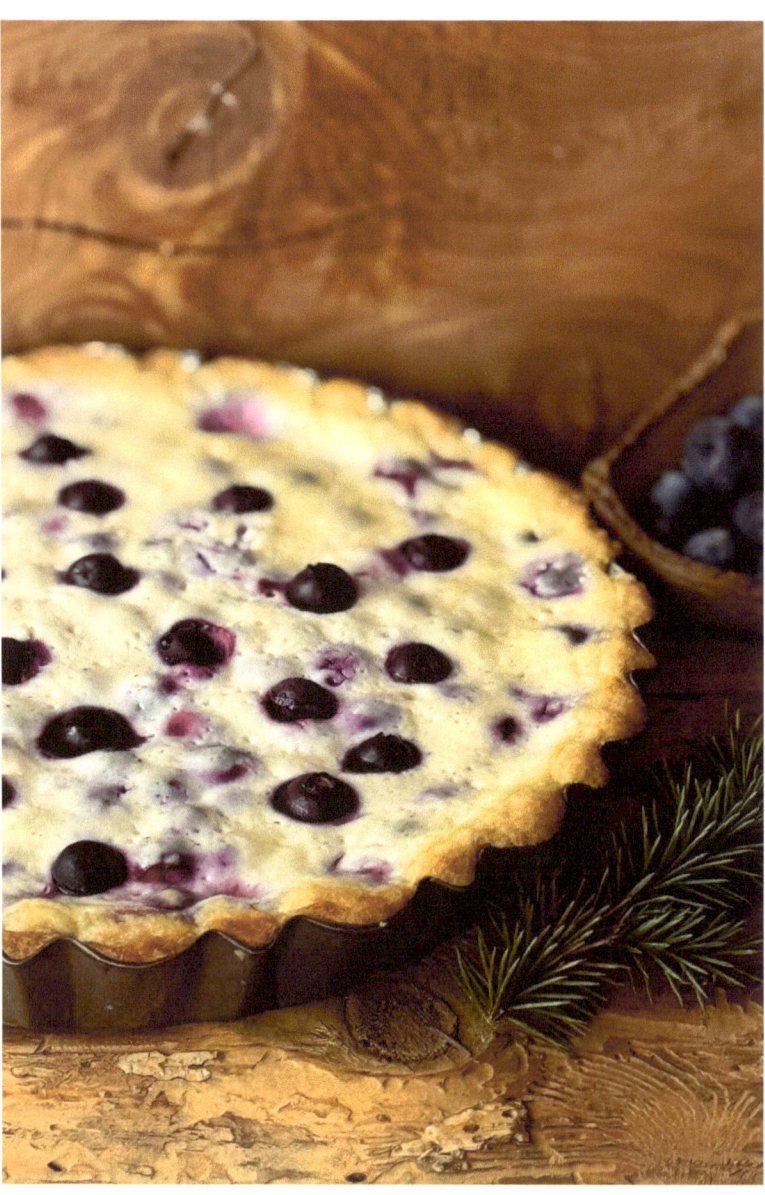

INGREDIENTS

For the Crust:

½ cup (116 g) unsalted butter

⅔ cup (130 g) sugar

1 egg

½ teaspoon vanilla

1 ¼ cups (155 g) all-purpose flour

1 teaspoon baking powder

¼ teaspoon cardamom

¼ teaspoon salt

For the Filling:

1⅓ cups (320 g) sour cream

1 egg

½ cup (100 g) sugar

¼ teaspoon cardamom

1 teaspoon vanilla

2 cups (12 oz) blueberries

DIRECTIONS

1. Preheat oven to 350°F (177°C). Lightly grease the tart pan if desired for easier removal.

2. In a stand mixer (or with an electric hand mixer) cream the butter and sugar on medium speed until pale color and light and fluffy (about 2 minutes). Add the egg and vanilla to the mixing bowl and beat until well combined, scraping down sides of the mixing bowl as you go.

3. In a bowl, whisk together the flour, baking powder, cardamom and salt. Working on low speed, add the flour mixture to the mixing bowl and beat until just combined. Do not overmix or the crust will be hard.

4. Gather the dough together and place it in the middle of the tart pan. Flour your hands and start working the dough outward so that it covers the bottom of the pan and goes up the sides of the pan to the top. You may have to re-flour your hands several times as the dough is quite sticky.

5. In a bowl or the clean mixer bowl, beat together the sour cream, egg, sugar, cardamom and vanilla until creamy and pourable.

6. Reserve about ¼ cup of blueberries and sprinkle the rest of them into the tart crust in one even layer. Pour the sour cream mixture on top of the blueberries, smoothing out with a spatula so that all blueberries are covered. Sprinkle the reserved blueberries on top of the batter.

7. Place the tart pan on a sheet pan to catch any drippings and make it easier to lift in and out of the oven. Bake for 35-45 minutes, or until edges of crust are golden brown and the center of the tart is set (it will firm up more after cooling). There may be some cracks in the top of the tart, similar to a cheesecake, but it will still be great.

8. Cool for several hours and then release the clasp on the side of the tart pan and gently lift the pan, removing it from the tart which remains on the bottom of the pan. Cover with aluminum foil or plastic wrap and refrigerate for up to 3 days. Serve cool or at room temperature.

SUBSTITUTIONS & ADDITIONS

- This Finnish pie is typically made with bilberries (similar to a wild blueberry) which are more abundant in Finland.

- The traditional dairy filling ingredient is a thick curd cream called Kermaviili. As this is not a common ingredient in North America, I used sour cream. Some recipes call for a mix of crème fraîche and sour cream.

- The traditional flour used for this pie in Finland is a rye flour, whereas this recipe uses all-purpose flour. You could also substitute a mix of all-purpose flour and wheat flour.

Nutrition Notes (per slice): Calories 375; Protein 9g; Carbs 41g; Fat 20g; Sugar 28g

MODERATE – Makes a 9 x 13" sheet cake (24 servings)

Chocolate Sheet Cake with Blueberry Cream Cheese Frosting

Keeping it easy does not always equal loss of flavor and texture, and this tender, rich, velvety sheet cake proves the point . I made a few simple modifications to a store-bought box cake (butter for oil and milk for water) and the results were très magnifique! The natural purple tones of the blueberry cream cheese frosting brought this simple cake up to company fare. No need for a fussy layer cake for a celebration dessert!

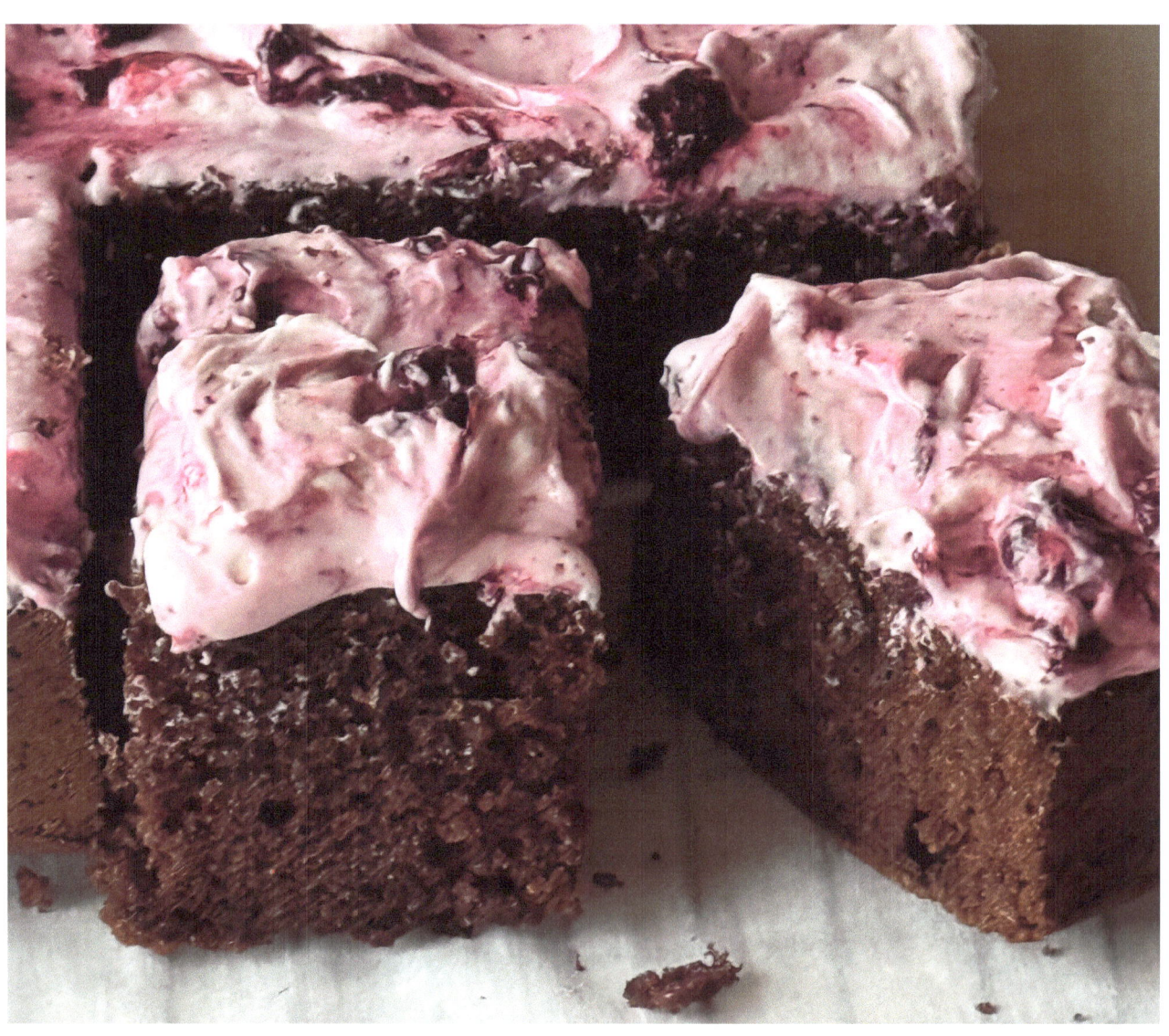

INGREDIENTS

For the Cake:

15.25 oz Duncan Hines "Perfectly Moist Devil's Food Chocolate Cake Mix"

1 cup (236 ml) whole milk, room temp.

3 eggs, room temp.

½ cup (113 g) unsalted butter, softened to almost melted

For the Frosting:

2 cups (12 oz) blueberries (I use frozen)

3 tablespoons sugar

1 tablespoon cornstarch

1 tablespoon lemon zest (grated zest from 1 medium lemon)

8 oz (226 g) full fat brick cream cheese (not a cream cheese spread), room temp.

½ cup (113 g) unsalted butter, room temp.

3 ¼ cups (375 g) powdered sugar

1 teaspoon vanilla

¼ teaspoon kosher salt

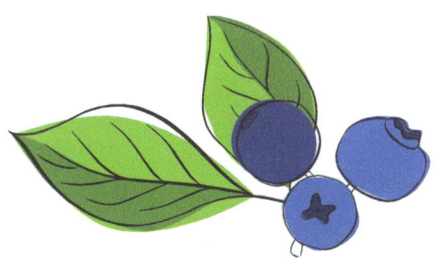

DIRECTIONS

For the Cake:

1. Preheat oven to 350°F (177°C). Spray bottom and sides of a 9 x 13" pan with cooking spray and set aside.

2. In a stand mixer or with an electric hand mixer, beat together the cake mix, milk, eggs and butter on medium speed for about 2 minutes, scraping the sides of the mixer bowl as needed.

3. Pour batter into the pan and bake for 26-31 minutes, or until a toothpick inserted in center of cake comes out clean. Cool completely in the pan before frosting.

For the Frosting:

4. First make a blueberry compote by combining blueberries, sugar, cornstarch and lemon zest in a saucepan and cooking over medium heat until the compote thickens (about 3-5 minutes). Remove from heat and set aside to cool.

5. While the compote is cooling, beat together the cream cheese and butter in a handheld or stand mixer on high speed. It should look creamy and smooth.

6. Add the powdered sugar (slowly to prevent flying out of the bowl), vanilla and salt and beat for 2 more minutes, scraping the sides as you go. If you prefer a thicker frosting, add a little more powdered sugar. Cover and refrigerate.

Assembly:

7. Make sure everything has cooled completely before assembly. Dollop spoonfuls of cream cheese frosting on the top of the cake and spread it around with a butter knife. Drop spoonfuls of compote onto the cream cheese frosting and swirl the compote into the cream cheese frosting with the tip of a clean butter knife. You may have some compote left over. Just keep it in the refrigerator covered and use on pancakes or waffles.

Nutrition Notes (per slice): 191 Calories; Protein 2g; Carbs 24g; Fat 11 ; Sugar 17g

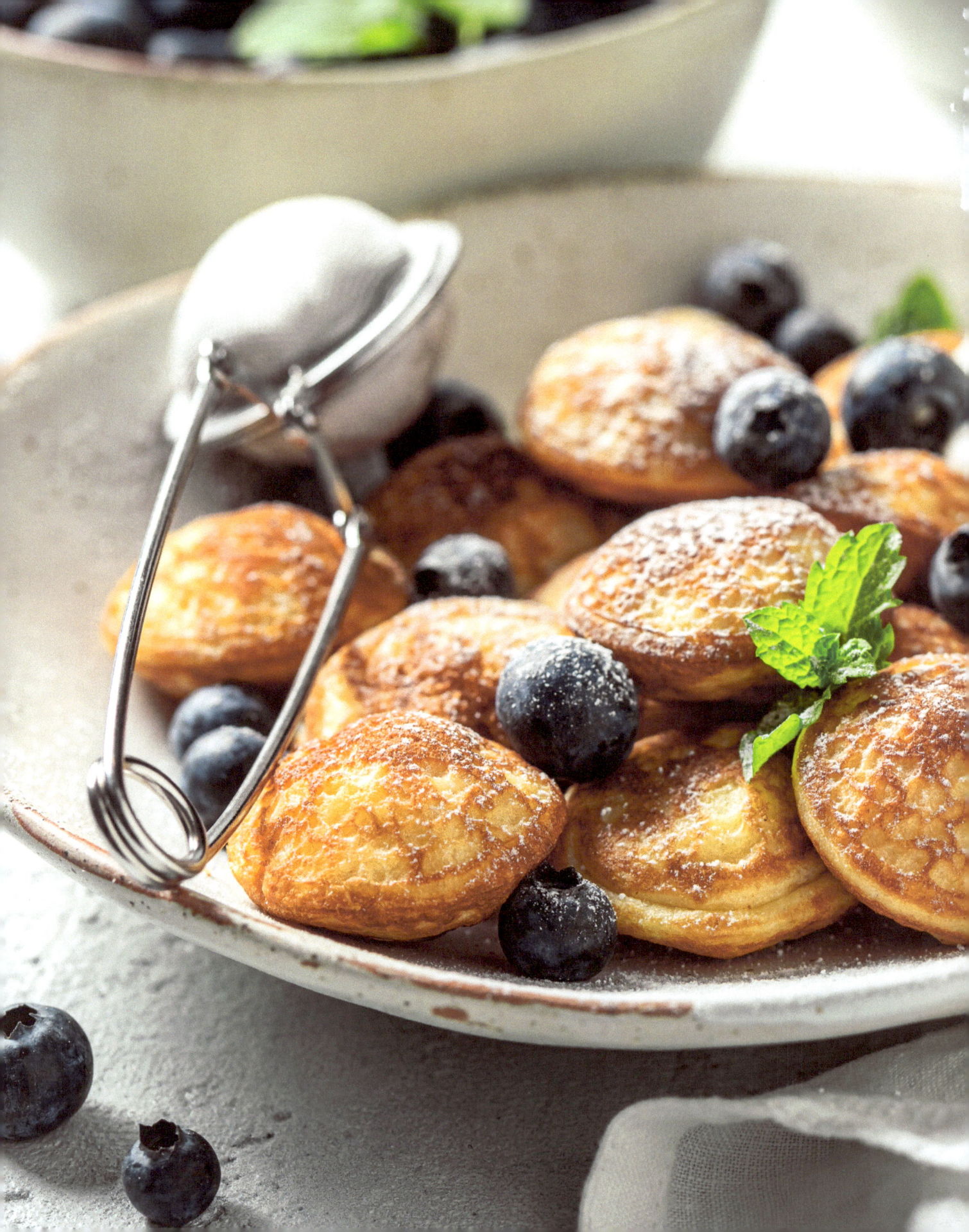

DIFFICULT — Serves 4 (4 large dinner plates)
Requires special equipment & 45 minute resting time

Poffertjes (Dutch Fair Food)

Poffertjes (pronounced POFF-ur-jis in English) are a classic fair food in the Netherlands (also known as Holland), and are as Dutch as tulips and windmills. They are similar to pancakes but much smaller, and airier due to the use of yeast. Food trucks at fairs and events serve them on paper plates, covered in melted butter and powdered sugar. They are a huge crowd-pleaser and every Dutch person's childhood favorite. This recipe serves them up with fresh blueberries or an easy blueberry compôte.

For the best results, you should really use a poffertjes pan. Traditionally made of cast iron, the most important characteristic of a poffertjes pan are the holes. This pan gives the poffertjes their typical fluffy round shape.

INGREDIENTS

1 cup white flour

1 cup buckwheat flour

1 tbsp white sugar

1 tbsp dry yeast; see notes

½ tsp salt

1.5 cups milk

1 egg

1.5 tbsp melted butter

COOKING NOTES

The use of yeast is what sets poffertjes apart from other pancakes. you can substitute baking powder for the yeast, but the result is always slightly off in my opinion.

DIRECTIONS

1. Mix the white flour, buckwheat flour, sugar, yeast and salt in a large mixing bowl.
2. Slowly mix in the milk, stirring continuously.
3. Add the egg and melted butter. Stir until you get a thick, well-mixed batter without lumps.
4. Cover the bowl and leave the batter to rest for 45 minutes in a warm location, so the yeast can do its work.
5. Once time is up, preheat your poffertjes pan on medium-high heat. Use the brush to grease it with some butter or your preferred type of oil.
6. Give the batter a last stir and pour it into a squeeze bottle or a piping bag with a small nozzle.
7. Squeeze batter in each of the holes in the pre-heated poffertjes pan, filling them to no more than ¾ of their capacity.
8. Cook over medium heat until bubbles start to form and the sides of the poffertjes have slightly solidified. Use a fork to quickly turn them. It can take some practice!
9. The poffertjes are done when they're golden brown on both sides. Serve with fresh blueberries or a blueberry compôte (see the Foundational Recipe chapter for a simple blueberry compôte).

Nutrition Notes (per 20-piece serving): Calories 83; Protein 3 g; Carbs 17 g; Fat 1 g; Sugar 6

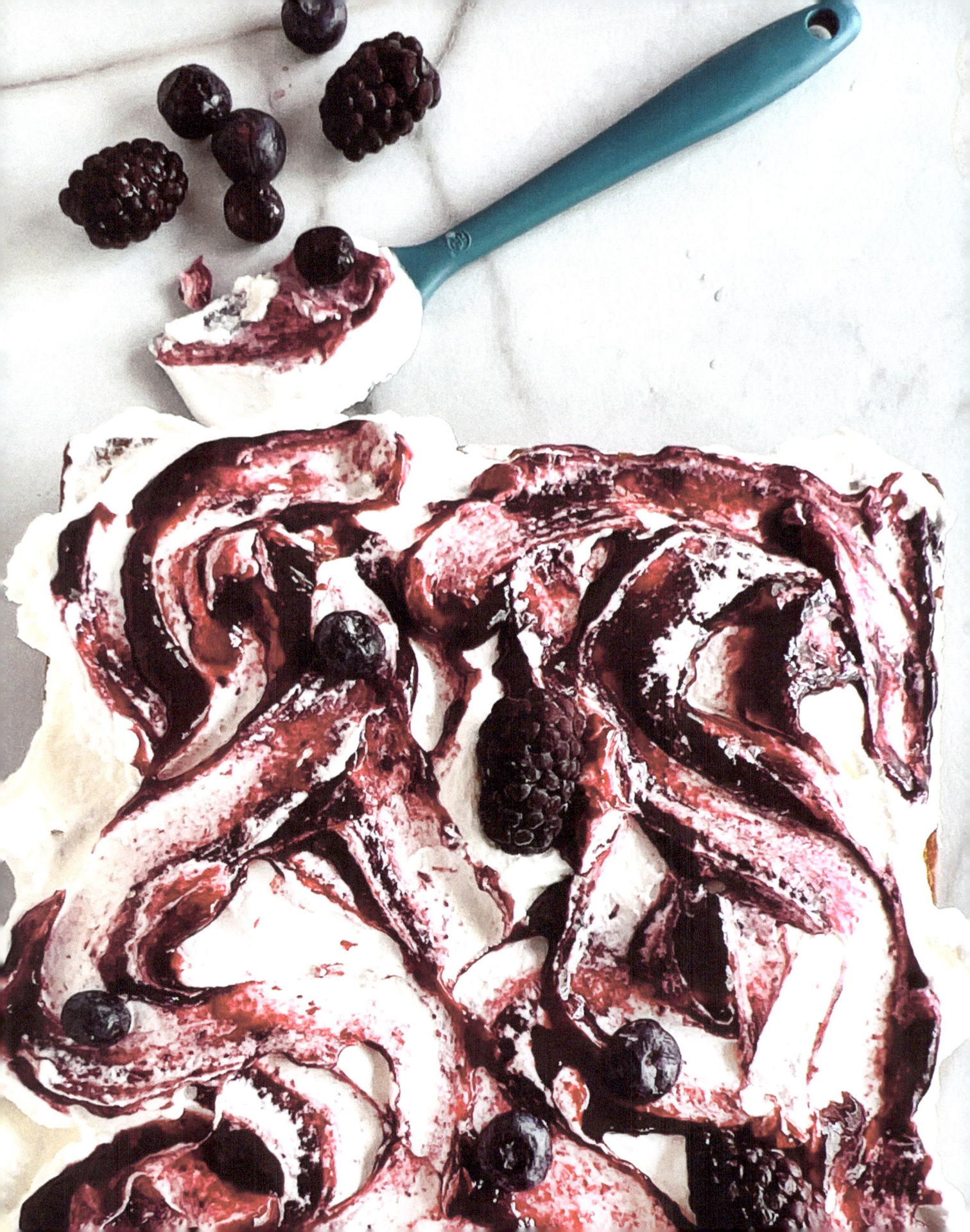

MODERATE – Makes a 9 x 13 dish (about 16 servings); Needs chilling time of 2+ hours

Blackberry-Blueberry Poke Cake

Poke cake is a retro dessert, traditionally made with boxed white cake mix, a tub of Cool-Whip and a box of Jell-O. It was introduced by a Jell-O advertisement in the 70's, and quickly became a favorite dish to take to a Midwestern potluck. There is no Jell-O or cool whip in this updated version, but also no need to make the cake from scratch. Keep the boxed cake mix, but make a fresh berry compote for the "pokes" and top it off with homemade lemon or vanilla whipped cream. Your retro potluck dish just got raves!

INGREDIENTS

1 box (15-18 oz) cake mix (white or yellow)

3 large eggs

1 ½ cups (9 oz) blueberries (can use frozen)

½ cup (3 oz) blackberries (can use frozen)

½ cup (100 g) granulated sugar

1 tablespoon cornstarch

⅛ teaspoon fine salt

2 teaspoons fresh lemon juice

2 cups (473 ml) fluid heavy cream

3 tablespoons powdered sugar

2 teaspoons vanilla extract

DIRECTIONS

For the Cake:

1. Preheat oven to 350°F (177°C).
2. Grease a 9 x 13 x 2-inch baking pan with cooking spray or butter.
3. With an electric mixer or stand mixer, mix the cake batter according to package directions, using the eggs listed above.
4. Bake for 35 minutes. Remove from oven and set aside.

For the Filling:

5. While the cake is baking, add blueberries, blackberries, sugar, cornstarch and salt to a medium saucepan and start cooking over medium-high heat. You can add a little water (maybe ½ cup) if the berries are too firm.
6. Bring to a boil and cook, stirring occasionally, for about 5 minutes. Reduce heat to medium and simmer until the mixture thickens and the berries begin to break down, about 8-10 minutes. If the blueberries did not break down and the filling is too chunky, let the filling cook and then transfer to a blender and blend until smooth and pourable. Stir in the lemon juice. Set aside.

Nutrition Notes (per serving): Calories 273; Protein 3g; Carbs 39g; Fat 13g; Sugar 23g

Make the "Pokes":

7. Allow the cake to cool slightly (about 10-15 minutes) and then begin poking the cake with the rounded end of a wooden spoon (or something similar that is rounded). Space the poke holes about 1 inch apart in rows with 2 inches between each row. This will result in 5 rows along the length of the pan and 4 pokes across the width. The holes should be deep enough where you almost hit the bottom of the pan.

8. Set aside ¼ of the berry filling to swirl in the whipped cream topping later. Spoon or drizzle the rest of the berry filling into the holes, filling each one up. After filling all holes, go back and refill any holes that need more with any remaining filling.

9. Cover and refrigerate the cake for at least 2 hours or overnight.

Final Assembly:

10. Prepare the whipped cream. In the bowl of a stand mixer fitted with the whisk attachment, combine the cream, sugar and vanilla and beat on medium speed until medium-stiff peaks form (about 5 minutes)

11. Generously top the cake with whipped cream. Place a small spoonful of reserved berry filling on the whipped cream topping and pull the spoon through it to leave berry swirls on top.

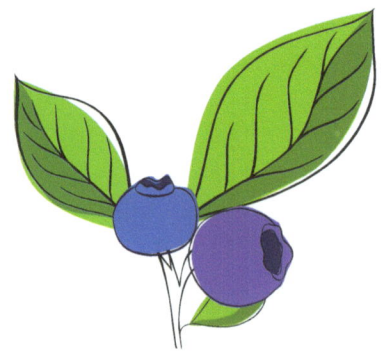

TO SHOW OFF THE POKES

- Part of the fun of a poke cake is to see the berry fillings when you first slice the cake. If you don't want to guess where to slice the cake, you will need to mark the location of the pokes. Before topping the cake with whipped cream, carefully remove the cake from the pan (this is the trickiest part).

- Use a small knife and make a vertical mark on the side of the cake in the location where a row of pokes lie. Those small marks will tell you where to slice for the visual appeal of seeing the "pokes". Otherwise you might just see a yellow cake with a whipped cream topping (which is not a bad thing).

- After the pokes are marked, generously top the cake with whipped cream (leaving the sides unfrosted so you can see the knife marks).

- When ready to slice the cake, check the sides where you marked the center of the location of the holes and slice along the rows of holes and serve. It makes for a really festive presentation!

SUBSTITUTIONS & ADDITIONS

- Strawberries are a popular berry to sub in for the blueberries.

- Another popular filling for the pokes is a salted caramel sauce.

- White, yellow or lemon cake have the most visual appeal when using blueberries for the "pokes".

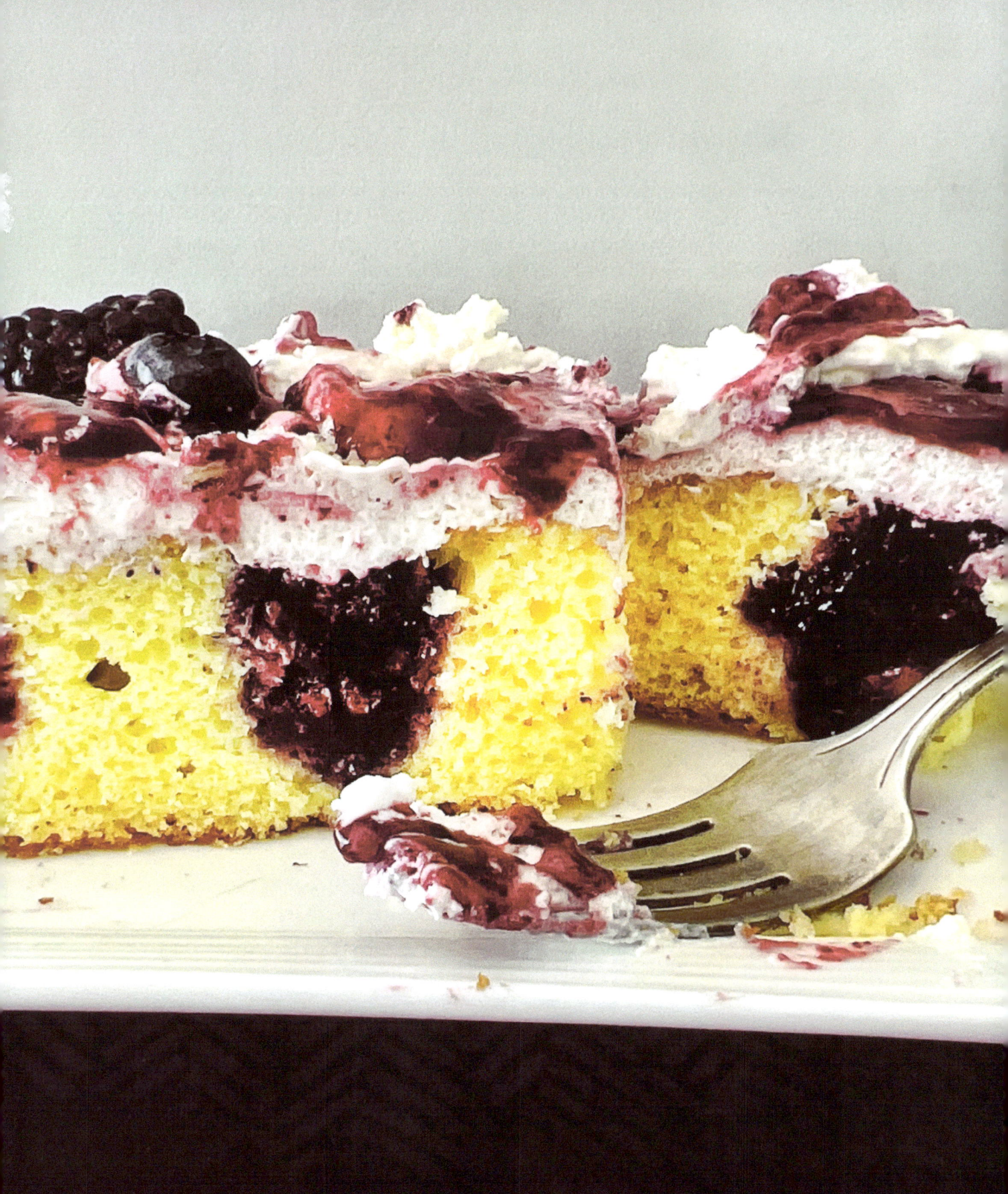

DIFFICULT — Makes 6 ¾-cup ramekins (serves 6)

Lemon Blueberry Soufflé

I have such fond memories of those warm, decadent chocolate pudding cakes from the casino buffets my grandparents frequented. I went in search of a lemon version of this type of dessert, but it took more trials than I anticipated before hitting the jackpot (so to speak). Most of my attempts ended up being more cake and less pudding than I wanted.

I finally landed on a combination of a lemon souffle and lemon pudding atop a jammy bed of blueberries inspired by Bon Appetit. Perfect! The puff layer of a souffle can be tricky, but I was shooting for a light cake topping rather than a tall puff. Each bite of this luscious dessert gives you a taste of a light cake, a tart lemon pudding, and a sweet layer of blueberry jam. It's not often that my home recipe ends up better than my food memory, but this one delivered!

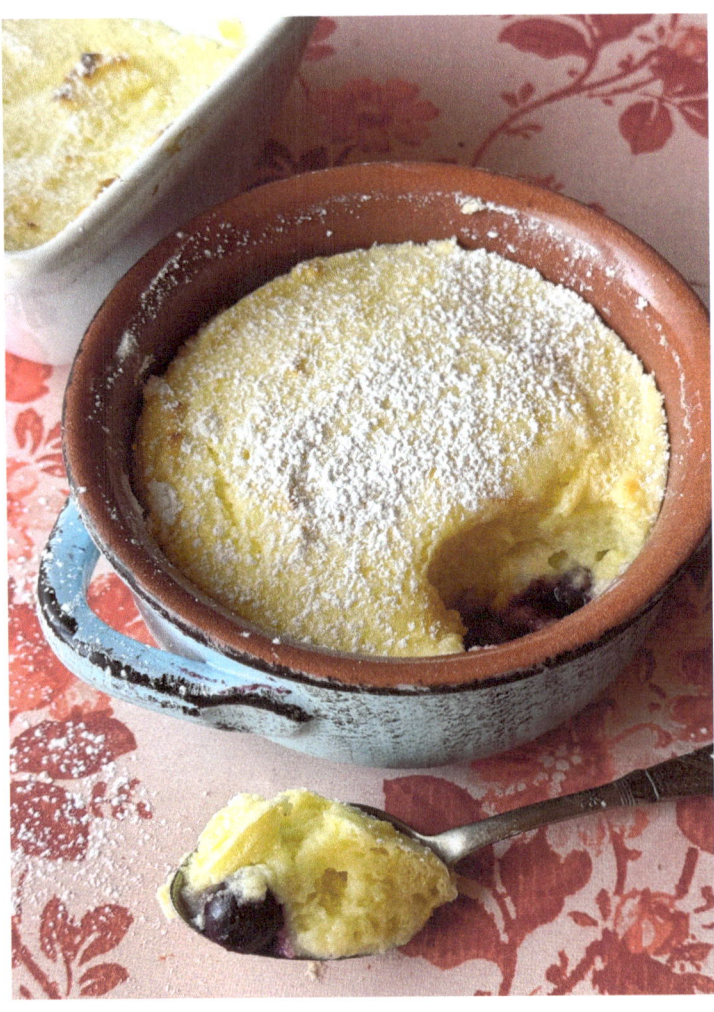

INGREDIENTS

3 large eggs, room temp.; yolks and whites separated

6 teaspoons blueberry jam

½ cup (3 oz) fresh or frozen blueberries

¾ cup (150g) sugar, divided into ½ cup and ¼ cup portions

2 tablespoons lemon zest

1 tablespoon cornstarch

¾ cup (185 ml) whole milk

2 tablespoons (¼ stick) unsalted butter, room temp

½ cup (118 ml) fresh lemon juice (about 3 large lemons)

⅛ teaspoon salt

Powdered sugar for garnish (optional)

DIRECTIONS

1. Preheat oven to 400°F (204°C). Prepare the ramekins by greasing them with a little softened butter and then sprinkling a bit of sugar evenly in the ramekins (tap them and turn upside down to distribute sugar).
2. Separate egg yolks from the whites into two small bowls. Set aside.
3. Spread jam on bottom of ramekins and distribute blueberries evenly on top of jam (about 4-5 blueberries per ramekin). Place ramekins on top of a large flat baking sheet.
4. In a medium saucepan, use a fork to press the lemon zest into the ½ cup of sugar to release the oils. Heat over low heat for 1 minute. Whisk in cornstarch until smooth, then gradually whisk in milk and egg yolks. Add butter and increase heat to medium, whisking continuously until mixture comes to a boil.
5. Continue whisking and boil for about 1 minute until a thick pudding forms.
6. Remove from heat and transfer to a large bowl so that it cools slightly. Stir the lemon juice and the salt into the bowl.
7. Using a stand mixer or electric hand mixer, beat reserved egg whites to soft peaks (whites will mound but no sharp tips will form). Gradually beat in reserved ¼ cup sugar. Beat until stiff but not dry. Peaks should be glossy and hold their shape (but not look grainy or curdled).
8. Using a spatula, gently fold whites into warm pudding with a cutting and turning motion, being careful not to deflate the whites. Spoon mixture over the berries, filling to the top of each ramekin.
9. Bake until slightly puffed and golden around the edges, about 12-16 minutes. Sift powdered sugar over the top and enjoy!

COOKING NOTES

Allow ingredients to come to room temperature for better success.

Some cooks will bake these in a water bath, which will allow more stable cooking throughout. If you want to use a water bath:

- place your ramekins in a large roasting pan;
- heat a pan of water on the stove to a boil;
- place roasting pan with dishes in oven and carefully pour hot water into pan around the dishes (about half way up the dishes).
- This method will take a little longer to cook so you will need to check frequently after 14 minutes.

Nutrition Notes: Calories 218; Protein 4g; Carbs 35g; Fat 7g; Sugar 32g

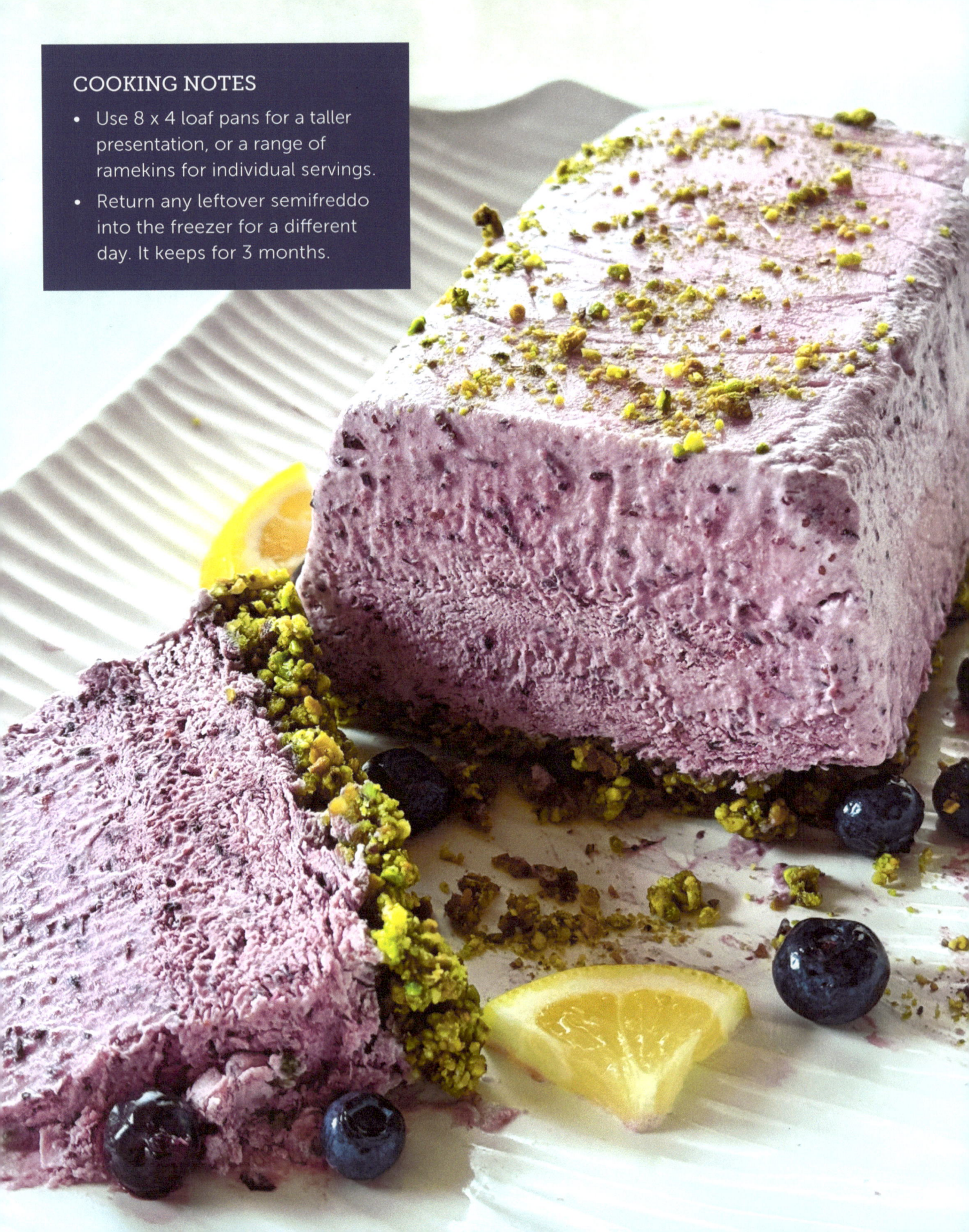

COOKING NOTES

- Use 8 x 4 loaf pans for a taller presentation, or a range of ramekins for individual servings.
- Return any leftover semifreddo into the freezer for a different day. It keeps for 3 months.

🥄🥄🥄 DIFFICULT — Makes two 9 x 5 x 2 ½-inch loaf pans (20 servings); Needs 3-4 hours chill time

Semifreddo: No Churn Ice Cream Dessert

Skip the pricey, bulky ice cream maker. This semifreddo is easier, tastes better, and only looks fancy—the hardest part is lining the pan. A refreshing summer dessert, with freezer-ready leftovers for later.

• •

INGREDIENTS

3 ½ cups (21 oz) blueberries

½ cup (112 g) granulated sugar

¾ cup (305 g) plain Greek yogurt

2 teaspoons lemon zest

1 teaspoon fresh lemon juice

¼ teaspoon vanilla

1 teaspoon balsamic vinegar

⅛ teaspoon salt

1 ¾ cups (412 ml) heavy whipping cream (cold)

1 ½ cups (185 g) crushed pistachio nuts

3 tablespoons unsalted butter, melted

DIRECTIONS

1. Line two 9 x 5 x 2 ½-inch loaf pans (or comparable volume dishes) with plastic wrap, leaving some to hang over edges

2. In a food processor, puree blueberries, sugar, Greek yogurt, lemon zest, lemon juice, vanilla, balsamic vinegar, and salt until smooth.

3. Beat heavy cream with a mixer until soft peaks form (peaks that will droop but still stand up by themselves).

4. Using a spatula, gently fold the blueberry mixture into the whipped cream until most streaks disappear. Don't overmix or you'll deflate the cream.
Fill pans to ¼ inch from top, cover with plastic, and freeze until mostly firm (≈1½ hours).

5. While the semifreddo freezes, crush pistachios with a mallet or food processor into fine crumbs. Microwave butter for about 25 seconds, then mix with the crumbs.

6. Remove semifreddo from freezer when firm and remove the plastic wrap on the top (not the plastic lining the inside). Distribute the nut crumb mixture over the top of each loaf, reserving ¼ cup for garnishing the top of the finished semifreddo. Cover the tops again and place back in the freezer for 2-3 hours.

7. When ready to serve, remove the top plastic wrap and turn the loaves upside down onto a plate. Run your hands along the outside and bottom of the pan to warm the metal enough to release from the pan.

8. Remove the rest of the plastic wrap and let soften for 5-10 minutes. Sprinkle with reserved nut crumb and slice into ¾ inch slices to serve.

Nutrition Notes (per serving): Calories 178; Protein 3g; Carbs 12g; Fat 14g; Sugar 9g

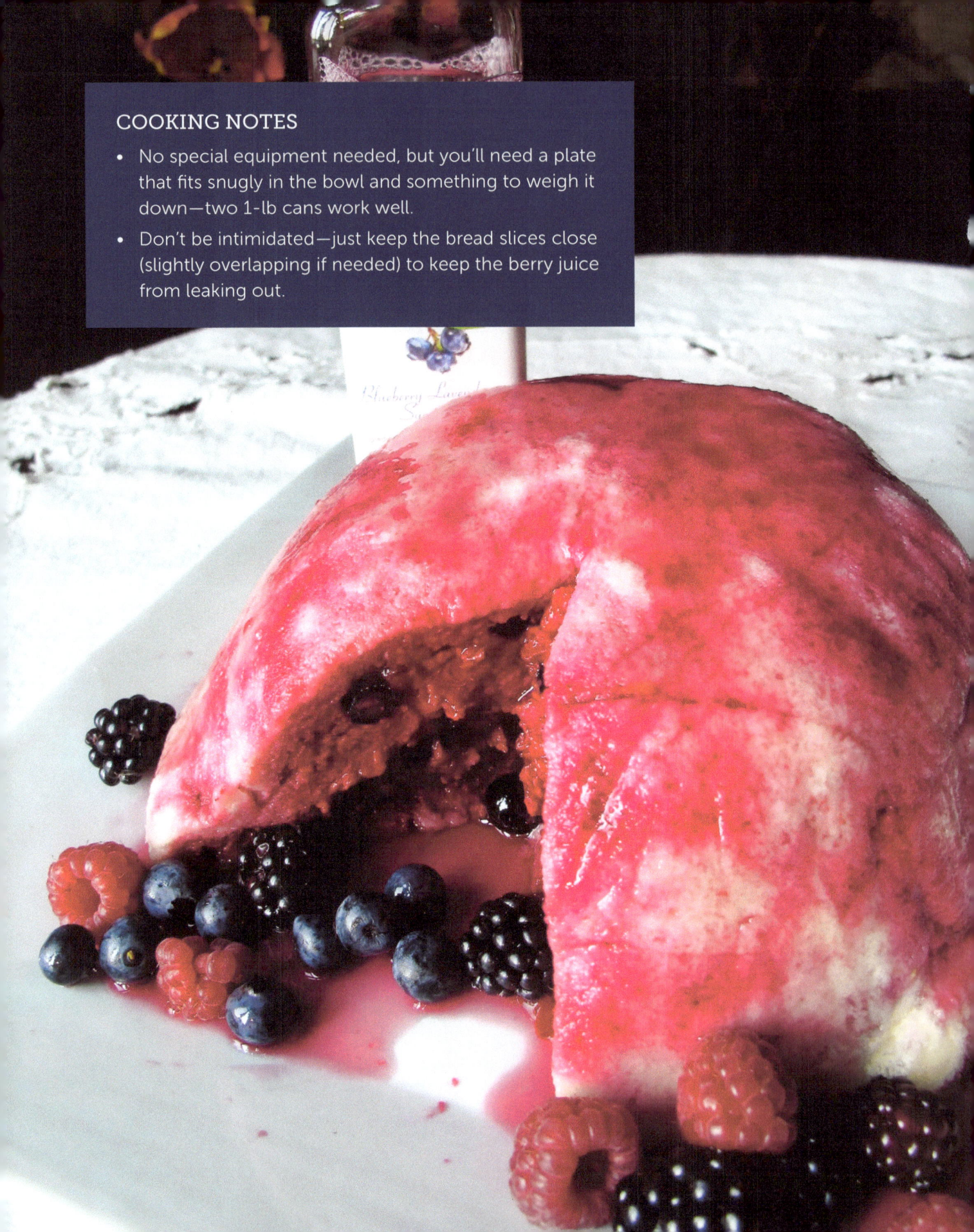

COOKING NOTES

- No special equipment needed, but you'll need a plate that fits snugly in the bowl and something to weigh it down—two 1-lb cans work well.
- Don't be intimidated—just keep the bread slices close (slightly overlapping if needed) to keep the berry juice from leaking out.

🥄🥄🥄 **DIFFICULT** — Makes 1 9-inch diameter bowl (about 8 servings); Needs overnight chilling

English Summer Pudding

The name summer pudding is rather a misnomer if you're from the States, as it isn't what Americans think of as pudding at all. To the British, the term pudding seems to cover everything from steamed savory dishes to molded cakes. This particular recipe for "summer pudding" is a classic English dessert made with seasonal berries inside of a soft white bread mold. It's deceptively easy to make, although it does take some forethought as it needs to chill overnight.

INGREDIENTS

2 ½ cups (14-16 oz) raspberries

1 ½ cups (9 oz) blackberries

1 ½ cups (9 oz) blueberries

1 ½ tablespoons Chambord liqueur

½ cup (150 g) sugar for cooking

12 slices firm white sandwich bread (Brioche is nice)

4 tablespoons sugar for use in layers

Mixed fresh berries for garnish

Whipped cream (optional)

DIRECTIONS

1. Combine the berries, Chambord, and sugar in a medium saucepan and cook over low heat for 2 minutes, or until sugar has dissolved. Remove pan from heat and set aside.
2. Trim crusts from bread and cut into diagonal halves (about 24 triangles).
3. Line a medium size bowl (about 1 ½ quarts or 9-inch diameter) with plastic wrap, allowing generous overhang on the sides.
4. Arrange 12–18 bread triangles in the bottom and up the sides, slightly overlapping to prevent leaks.
5. With a slotted spoon, add half the berries to the bread-lined bowl, sprinkle with 2 Tbsp sugar, and cover with 2 bread slices.
6. Top with remaining berries, 2 Tbsp sugar, and 2–3 bread triangles, leaving no gaps. Reserve any remaining juice from the fruit and set aside.
7. After covering the fruit with bread, fold the overhanging plastic wrap over the top. Place a plate (that fits inside the bowl) on top, weigh it down with 2 heavy cans or a 2-lb weight, and refrigerate for at least 8 hours or overnight.
8. To serve, remove the weight and the plate and unfold the plastic wrap that covered the top. Let the rest of the plastic wrap hang over the sides. Place a large plate on top of the bowl and flip it over. Gently lift off the bowl and peel away wrap.
9. Slice with a sharp knife and garnish with fresh berries or mint.

Nutrition Notes (per serving): Calories 157; Protein 5g; Carbs 30g; Fat 2g; Sugar 9g

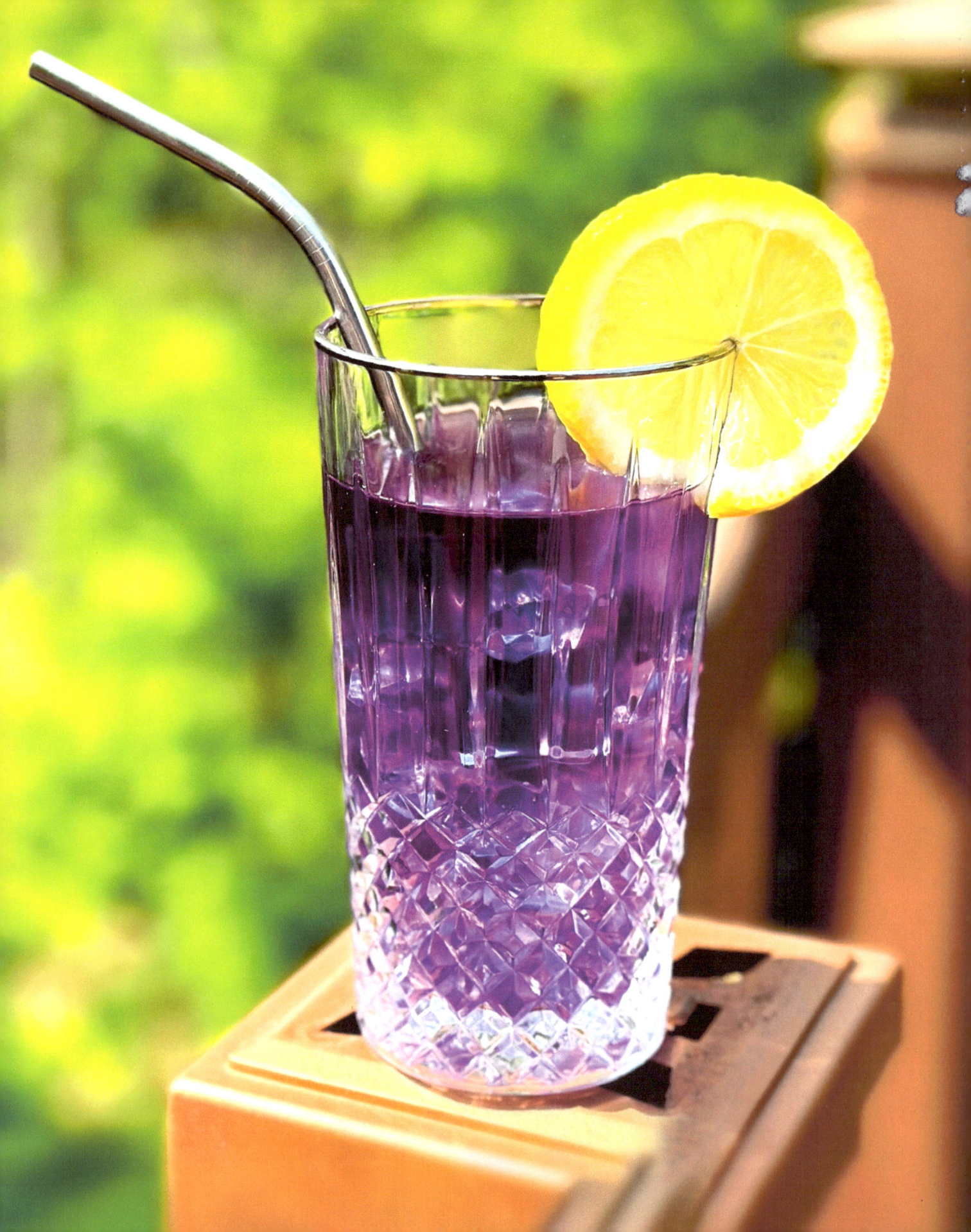

DRINKS

Basil Lemonade

Italian Sodas/Spritzers

Cocktails: Martini & Mojito

Looseleaf Tea
with Dried Blueberries

Blueberry Raspado
(Mexican Shaved Ice)

Mexican Berry Atole

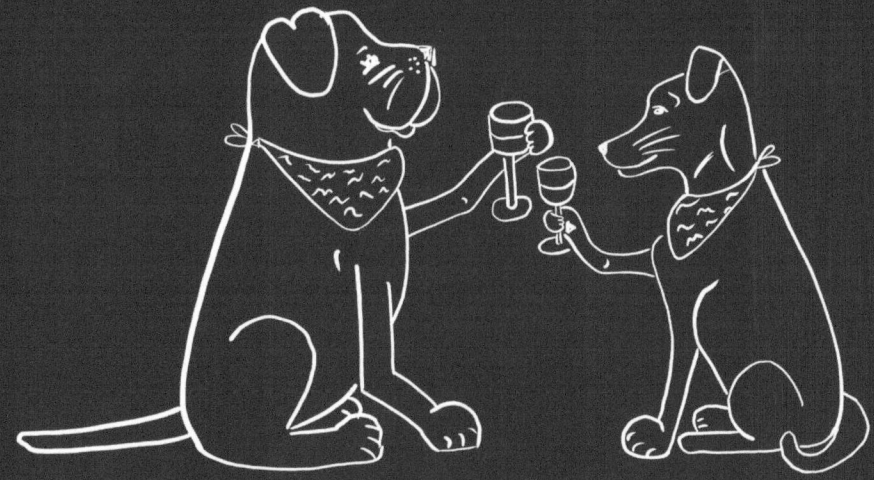

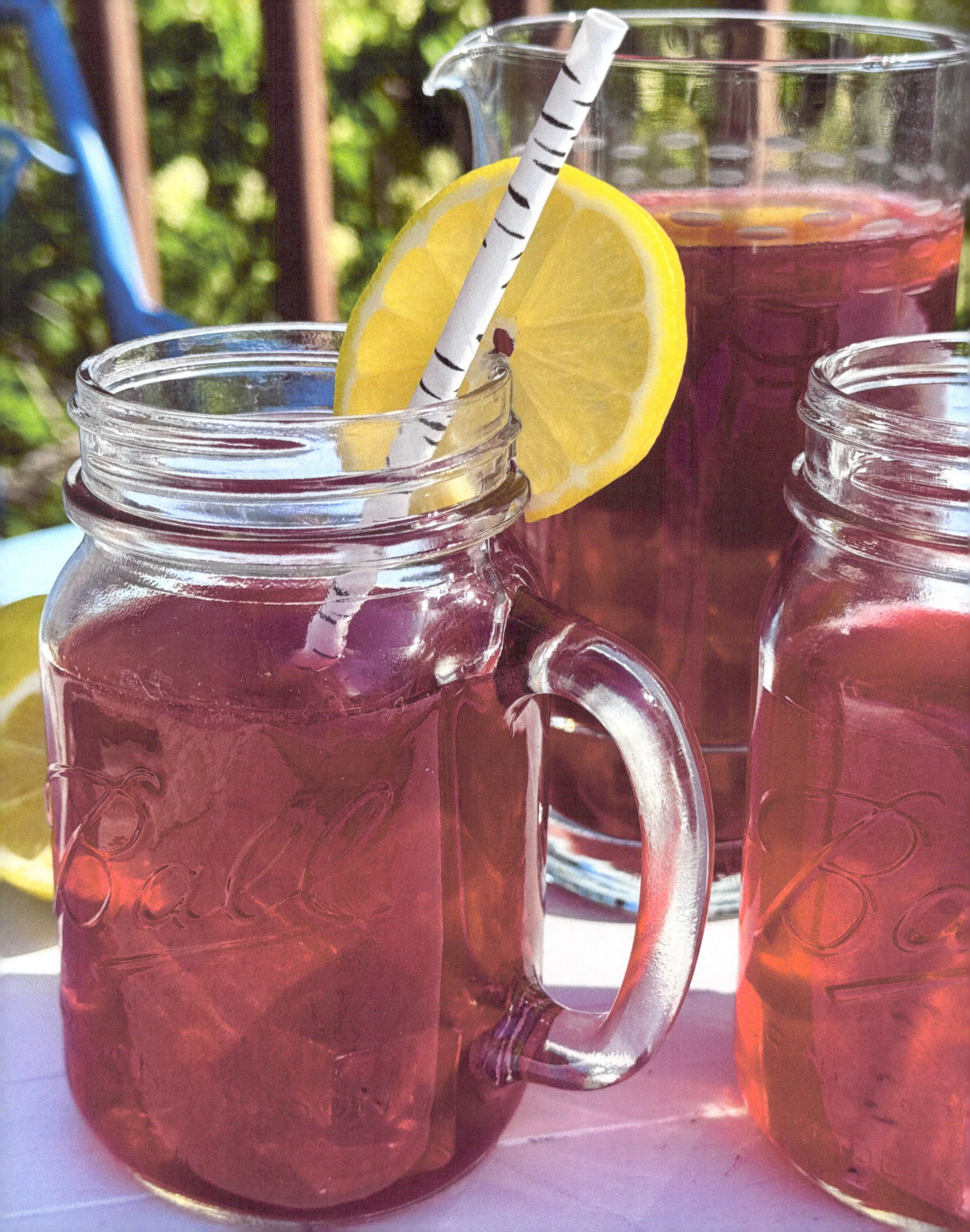

EASY — Makes 6 tall glasses

Basil Lemonade

My favorite vendor at the St. Paul farmers' market sells bagel sandwiches and fresh squeezed lemonade. He has been there since 1998 and there is always a long line on those hot summer days for the lemonade. My booth happens to be right next to his, and as soon as the sun comes out, I'm at his stand for a refresher to keep me friendly for the rest of the market day.

This year I brought some of the blueberry juice from my drained frozen blueberries and added a little to his fresh lemonade for the best taste treat at market! He better watch out…my blueberry riff on his lemonade might just give him some competition!

INGREDIENTS

1 cup (237 ml) warm water (for blending)

¾ cup (150 g) sugar

1 cup (6 oz) blueberries

¼ cup whole basil leaves, packed

1 cup (237 ml) freshly squeezed lemon juice

¼ teaspoon salt

4 cups (946 ml) water (for mixing)

DIRECTIONS

1. In a blender, combine 1 cup warm water, sugar, blueberries, basil leaves, lemon juice, and salt. Process until combined (about 1 minute). Taste and stir in more sugar at this time if you want it sweeter.

2. Pour the mixture through a fine-mesh strainer into a bowl. Allow the juice to slowly drain without pushing it through the strainer if you want a clear juice. For pulpy juice, press mixture through a strainer with a spoon.

3. Add the blueberry-lemon mixture to a pitcher and stir in 4 cups of water. Chill. To serve, pour into ice-filled glasses.

SUBSTITUTIONS & ADDITIONS

- Substitute sparkling water for the still water for a bubbly lift.
- Substitute limes for the lemons for a tangy limeade.
- Instead of basil, infuse the blueberries with thyme or aromatic spices like star anise and cardamom.

Nutrition Notes (per glass): Calories 119; Protein 0.3g; Carbs 31g; Fat 0.3g; Sugar 28g

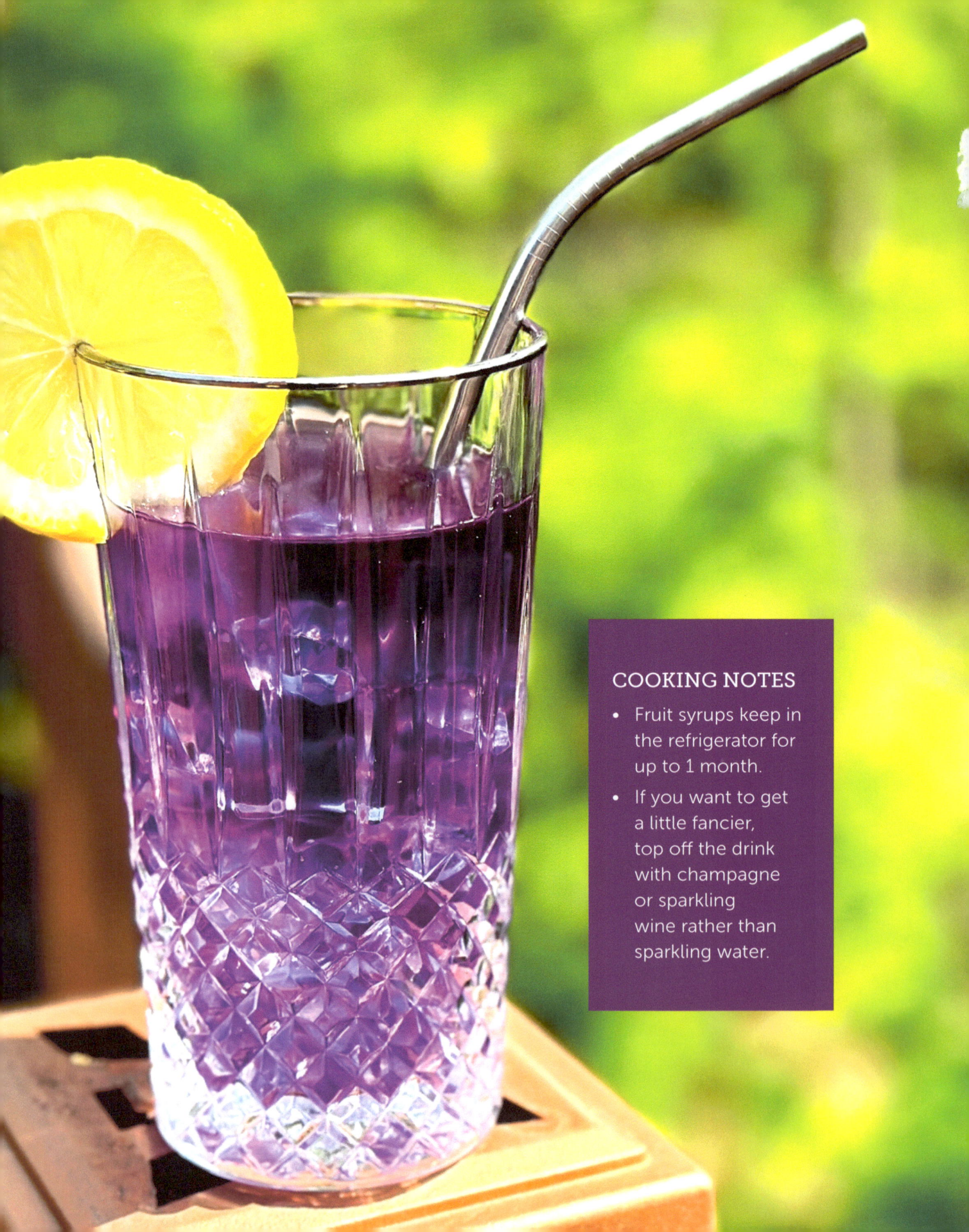

COOKING NOTES

- Fruit syrups keep in the refrigerator for up to 1 month.
- If you want to get a little fancier, top off the drink with champagne or sparkling wine rather than sparkling water.

🥄 *EASY — The syrup makes 1½ cup syrup (about 24 tablespoons)*

Italian Sodas/Spritzers

In an effort to put my decade of bartending experience together with my later decade(s) of farming experience, I developed a wide range of drink syrups which I sold at the farmers markets up until 2022. The easiest (and most popular) way that these syrups were used was in making Italian sodas (aka spritzers).

Italian sodas are essentially flavored syrups + carbonated water + fruit garnish. Once you make the fruit syrup you just fill a glass with club soda, sparkling water, or tonic water and stir in 2-3 Tablespoons of blueberry simple syrup. The secret to a "great" Italian soda however is using real fruit, no corn syrup and herbal or spice infusions in your simple syrup, all of which are hard to come by in commercial products. Once you try Italian sodas with your own fresh syrup, you will be hard pressed to have them any other way.

• •

INGREDIENTS

1 cup (200 g) granulated sugar

1 cup (237 ml) water

1 cup (6 oz) fresh blueberries

1 teaspoon lemon juice

¼ cup herbs or ⅛ cup whole spices
(optional, used for infusions)

For the Italian Soda:

2-3 tablespoons blueberry syrup

6-8 oz (177-237 ml) sparkling water (or club soda)

DIRECTIONS

For the Syrup:

1. In a small saucepan cook sugar and water over medium heat, stirring until sugar dissolves (about 2 minutes).

2. Stir in the blueberries and lemon juice. Add the herbs and/or spices at this time if you are making an infusion. Reduce heat to low and simmer for about 10 minutes, or until berries have burst. If you are doing a flavor infusion, remove the pan from the burner and allow the herbs or spices to steep in the pan for 20 minutes before straining.

3. Strain the berry mixture through a mesh sieve into a glass bottle with a lid or a covered stainless steel container.

For the Italian Soda:

Fill an 8-ounce glass with ice. Add 2 tablespoons of the simple syrup (recipe above) and fill the glass with sparkling water. Stir together and taste. Add another tablespoon of syrup if you want a sweeter drink. Garnish with a lemon peel or a sprig of mint (optional).

For a French soda:

Stir in 1-2 teaspoons of heavy cream.

Nutrition Notes (per tablespoon): Calories 4; Protein .05g; Carbs 1g; Fat .02g; Sugar 1g

🥄 EASY — Makes 1½ cup syrup (about 24 tablespoons)

Martinis & Mojitos Using Blueberry Syrup

There is no easier way to turn a standard cocktail (or mocktail) into something special than by using fruit drink syrups made with real, whole fruit. The difference between using a homemade drink syrup with real fruit in a cocktail rather than the commercial flavored syrups is something to behold. These are my 2 favorite cocktails using blueberry syrup.

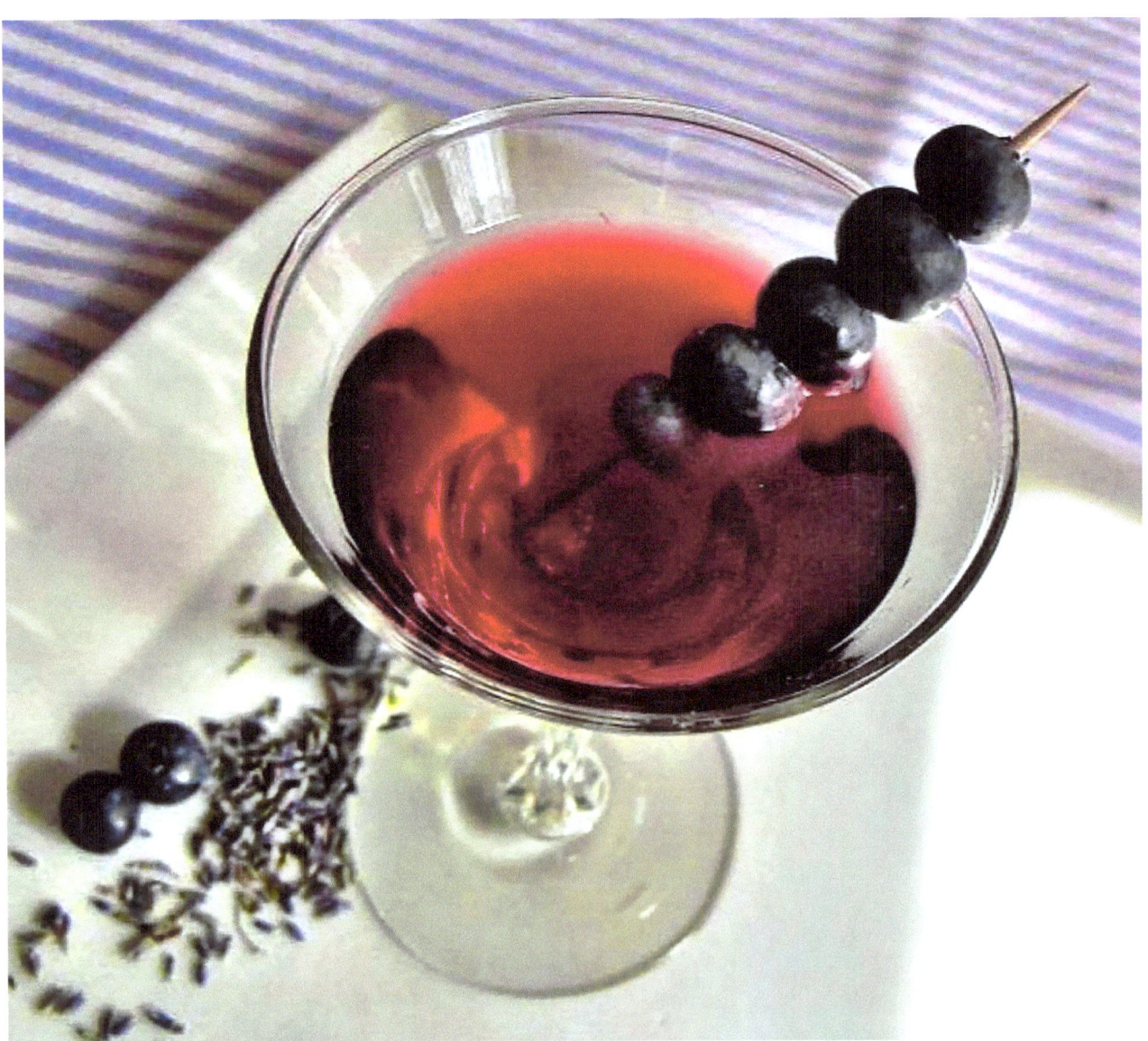

BLUEBERRY SIMPLE SYRUP

- In a small saucepan, cook 1 cup (200 g) sugar and 1 cup (237 ml) water over medium heat, stirring until sugar dissolves (about 2 minutes). Stir in 1 cup (6 oz) blueberries and reduce heat to low. Simmer for about 10 minutes, or until berries have burst.
- Strain the berry mixture through a mesh sieve into a glass bottle with a lid or a covered stainless steel container.

BLUEBERRY MARTINI

- Fill a shaker with ice cubes.
- Add 2 oz vodka or gin, 1 oz blueberry drink syrup, a dash of bitters and a squeeze of 1 lime wedge to shaker
- Shake well and strain into a chilled cocktail glass
- Garnish with fresh blueberries or another lime wedge

Nutrition Notes (per martini): Calories: 207; Protein 0; Carbs 19 g; Fat 0; Sugar 13 g

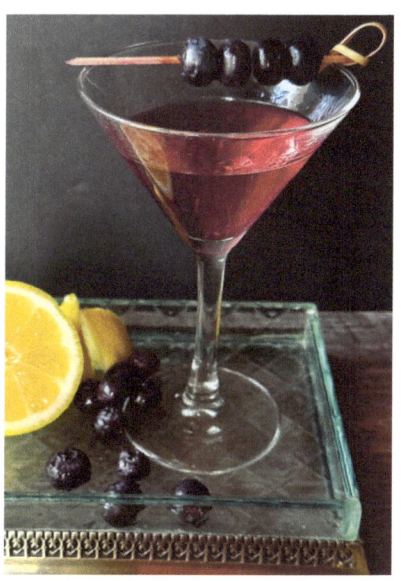

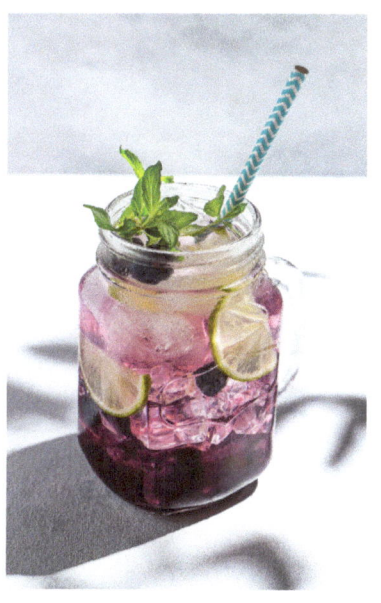

BLUEBERRY MOJITO

- Add ½ cup (3 oz) blueberries, 2 lime wedges and about 8 mint leaves to a cocktail shaker. Use a muddler to mash everything together. Muddle enough that the lime juice is released from the limes and the oils are released from the mint leaves. The mashed blueberries will still retain a pulpy texture.
- Add 3 tablespoons blueberry syrup and 2 oz rum to the shaker and stir together. Add ice to a glass and strain the mixture into the glass through the shaker's built in strainer.
- Top it off with sparkling water.

Nutrition Notes (per mojito): Calories: 370; Protein 1 g; Carbs 56 g; Fat 0.3; Sugar 51 g

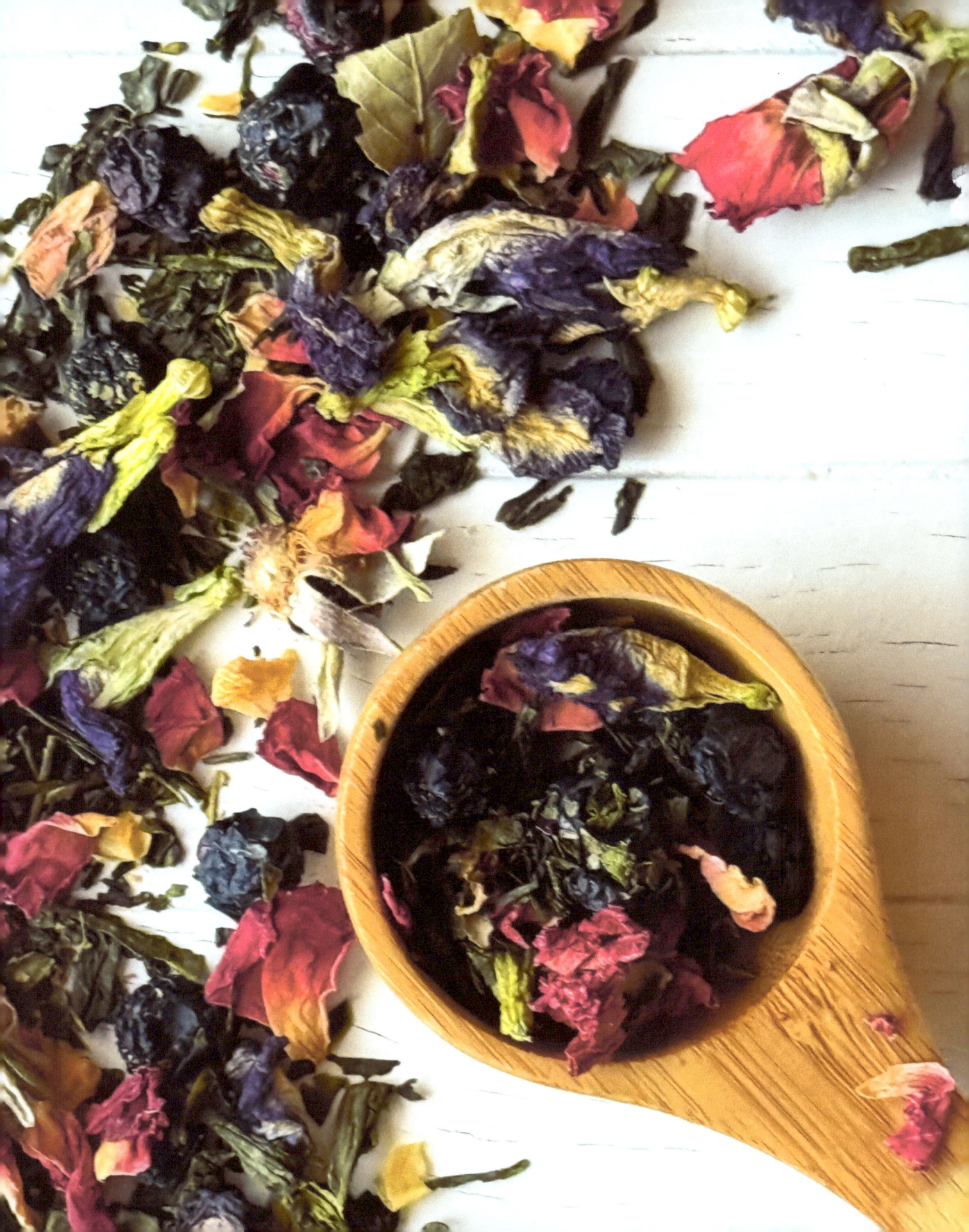

EASY — Makes about 25 cups of tea at 1 teaspoon per cup

Looseleaf Tea with Dried Blueberries

While blueberries are the major crop on our Minnesota farm, herbs come in at a close second. There are so many wonderful things to do with herbs (fresh and/or dried), but the way I use them the most is in blending herbal teas. I started blending teas as a way to address some personal health issues, and ended up doing a deep dive into the myriad health benefits associated with herbal teas.

Because green tea and blueberries both wear the health halo, I dried some blueberries and added them to some looseleaf green sencha tea, along with some dried ginger. It is my absolute favorite in terms of both flavor and health benefits. You can use this recipe as a template, but feel free to customize to your preferences.

This recipe is best understood in ratios instead of precise measurements, so that you can blend the amount that best suits you. I have listed the ingredients in terms of cups instead of weights, as volume is more relevant than weight when blending teas.

INGREDIENTS

½ cup looseleaf green tea

¼ cup dried blueberries

¼ cup dried ginger root

⅛ cup dried orange peels

SUBSTITUTIONS & ADDITIONS

- Mint is a popular flavor combination with blueberries. Substitute ¼ cup mint for ¼ cup ginger. Alternatively you can just add the mint along with the ginger.
- If you want a bright blue color for visual appeal, add ¼ cup Butterfly Pea flowers to the mixture. Butterfly Pea flowers have no taste, but they turn the tea into a blue-green color. When you add a lemon squeeze, something magical happens and the tea turns purple!

DIRECTIONS

1. In a large bowl, combine all ingredients and mix together thoroughly with your hands. Transfer to a sealable bag or container and keep in a cool dry place.

2. For a cup of hot tea: place 1-2 teaspoons in a small teapot (or a large tea ball) and steep at 160-175°F (71- 79°C) for 2-3 minutes. Do not steep green tea too hot or for too long or it will be bitter.

3. For iced tea: In a pitcher, stir together 3 tablespoons of tea and 6-8 cups (1.4-1.9 l) cold water. Refrigerate overnight and strain into a clean container when ready to serve.

Nutrition Notes (per cup of tea): Calories 14; Protein 0.3g; Carbs 3g; Fat 0.1g; Sugar 1g

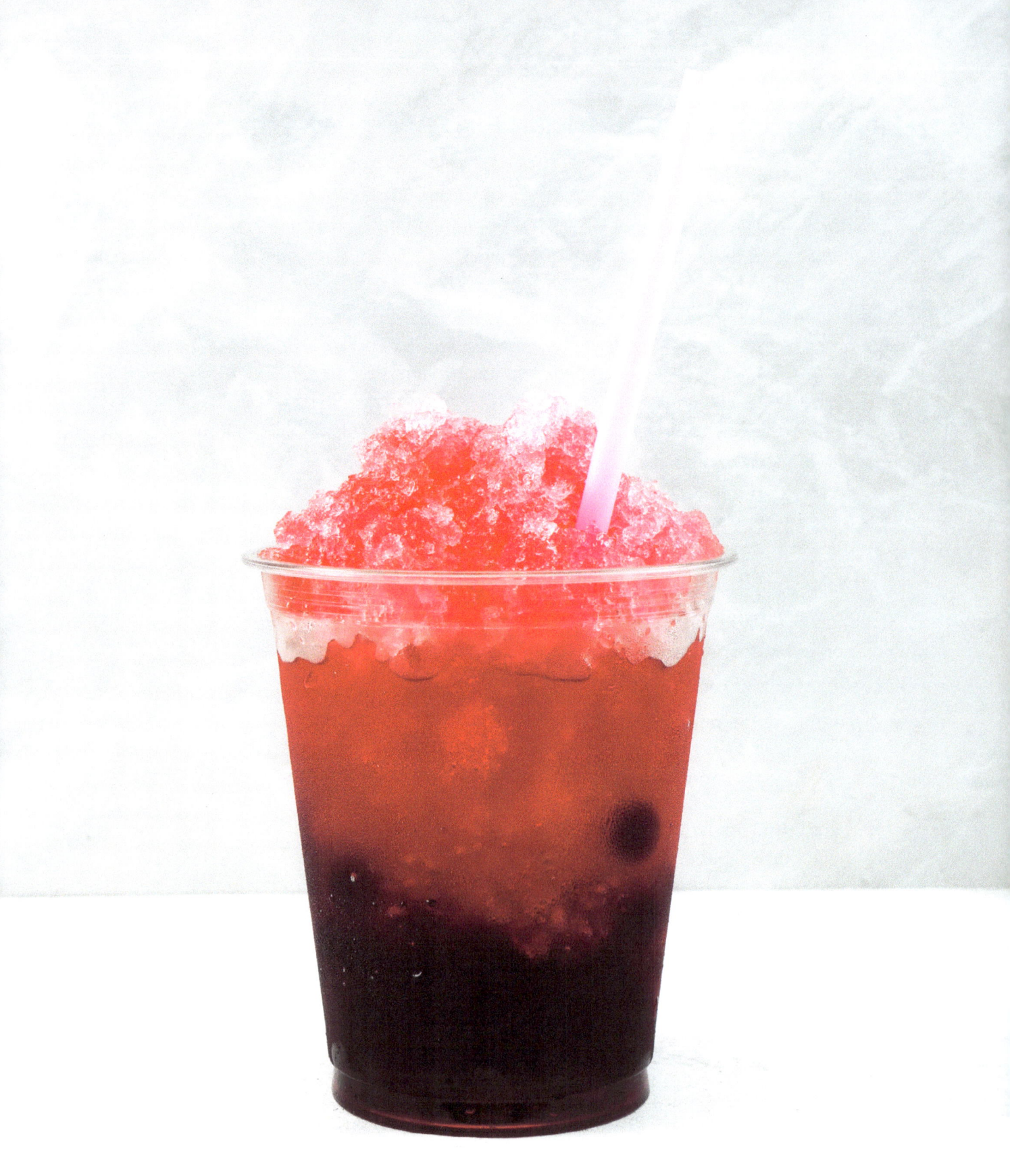

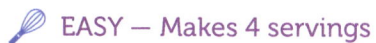 EASY — Makes 4 servings

Blueberry Raspado (Mexican Shaved Ice)

In many places in Mexico you will find street vendors with a huge block of ice and a colorful collection of flavored syrups, ready to delight customers with a refreshing sweet treat. They crush or scrape the ice with an "ice scratcher", scoop it into a cup, and then bathe the shaved ice in a natural, fruity syrup. If you have a blender at home, you too can make this delicious summer treat in less than an hour. No specialized equipment necessary!

INGREDIENTS

2 cups (473 ml) water

1 cup (200 g) granulated sugar

2 cups (12 oz) blueberries

8 cups ice

SUBSTITUTIONS & ADDITIONS

- Any fruity simple syrup will work but stick to natural flavors
- Top off your raspado with a sprinkle of chile lime seasoning (like Tajin)
- Add a little lime juice to the blueberry syrup once it cools.
- For a fun adults-only twist add a couple of ounces of tequila.
- For an extra-indulgent treat, drizzle in some sweetened condensed milk to mix with the blueberry syrup.

DIRECTIONS

1. Add the water and sugar to a medium saucepan and heat over medium-high, stirring until sugar dissolves (about 2 minutes).
2. Add the blueberries, reduce heat to medium and cook for 15-20 minutes, or until berries burst and the mixture is a thin syrup consistency. It's OK to have blueberry chunks in the syrup, but if you want a smoother syrup either strain the berry mixture or blend it until smooth. Allow the mixture to cool for at least 30 minutes, so as not to melt the ice.
3. When ready to serve, add 4 cups of ice cubes to a blender and blend until ice is finely crushed, like snow cone texture. Transfer crushed ice to a bowl and repeat with the remaining ice.
4. To assemble, divide the crushed ice among 4 cups or glasses and pour about ¼ cup of the blueberry syrup on top of each. Serve immediately.

COOKING NOTES

- The syrup makes about 3 cups, which is probably more than is needed for 4 servings. The leftover syrup will keep for up to a month, covered in the refrigerator and can be used for more raspados or other drinks (i.e., Italian sodas).
- Raspados melt pretty quickly, so make sure to put them together right before serving.
- Crushed ice does not store well, so it needs to be done at serving time.

Nutrition Notes: Calories 229; Protein 1g; Carbs 59g; Fat 1g; Sugar 55g

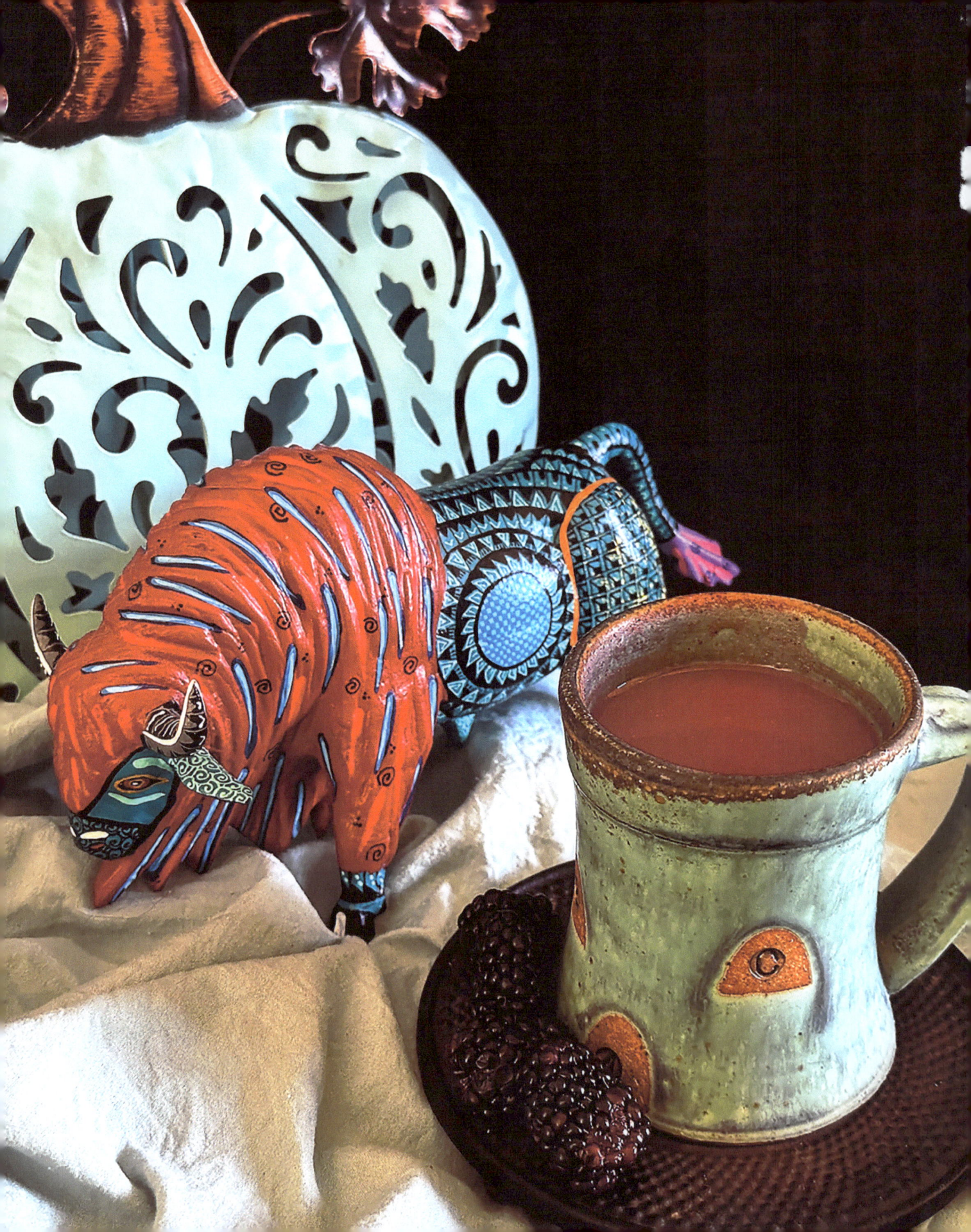

MODERATE – Makes 6 cups

Mexican Berry Atole

While on a recent trip to Oaxaca, I discovered atole—a traditional Mexican drink that was completely new to me but beloved throughout Mexico. Atole is a warm, comforting beverage thickened with masa harina and often served at breakfast as a liquid porridge. Atoles come in countless flavors—fruity, nutty, spicy, or the rich chocolate version called champurrado. My blueberry version brings American flavors to this ancient Mexican drink.

INGREDIENTS

4 cups (1 liter) water

2 whole star anise

2 whole allspice berries

⅓ cup (75 g) brown sugar (piloncillo if available)

¼ teaspoon kosher salt

2 cups (12 oz) blueberries (fresh or frozen)

1 cup (237 ml) cold water

¾ cup (93 g) masa harina (Maseca brand if available)

SUBSTITUTIONS & ADDITIONS

- Blackberries are a classic fruit for a Mexican atole, but you can substitute in any of your favorite berries
- Cinnamon is a good pairing with blueberries and can be substituted or added to the star anise or allspice berries (use cinnamon sticks rather than ground cinnamon).

DIRECTIONS

1. Add 4 cups water and spices to a large saucepan and bring to a boil. Turn off heat and let the spices infuse into the water for about 15 minutes. Remove the spices with a slotted spoon and discard.
2. Add the sugar and the salt to the pan and heat over medium heat, stirring, until the sugar is dissolved (2-3 minutes). Reduce heat to a low simmer.
3. To a blender, add blueberries, 1 cup of water and the masa and puree until very smooth. Pour the blended mixture through a fine-mesh strainer into the pan with the spiced water.
4. Simmer mixture over medium-low heat, stirring often with a wire whisk until mixture is thickened to a consistency similar to thin pudding (15-30 minutes). If it is lumpy, you may want to strain again.
5. Serve warm in mugs.

COOKING NOTES

Leftover atole will thicken quite a bit. You can store it in the refrigerator for up to 3 days, and then add a little water to the mixture when you reheat it.

Nutrition Notes (per cup): Calories 133; Protein 2g; Carbs 31g; Fat 1g; Sugar 20g

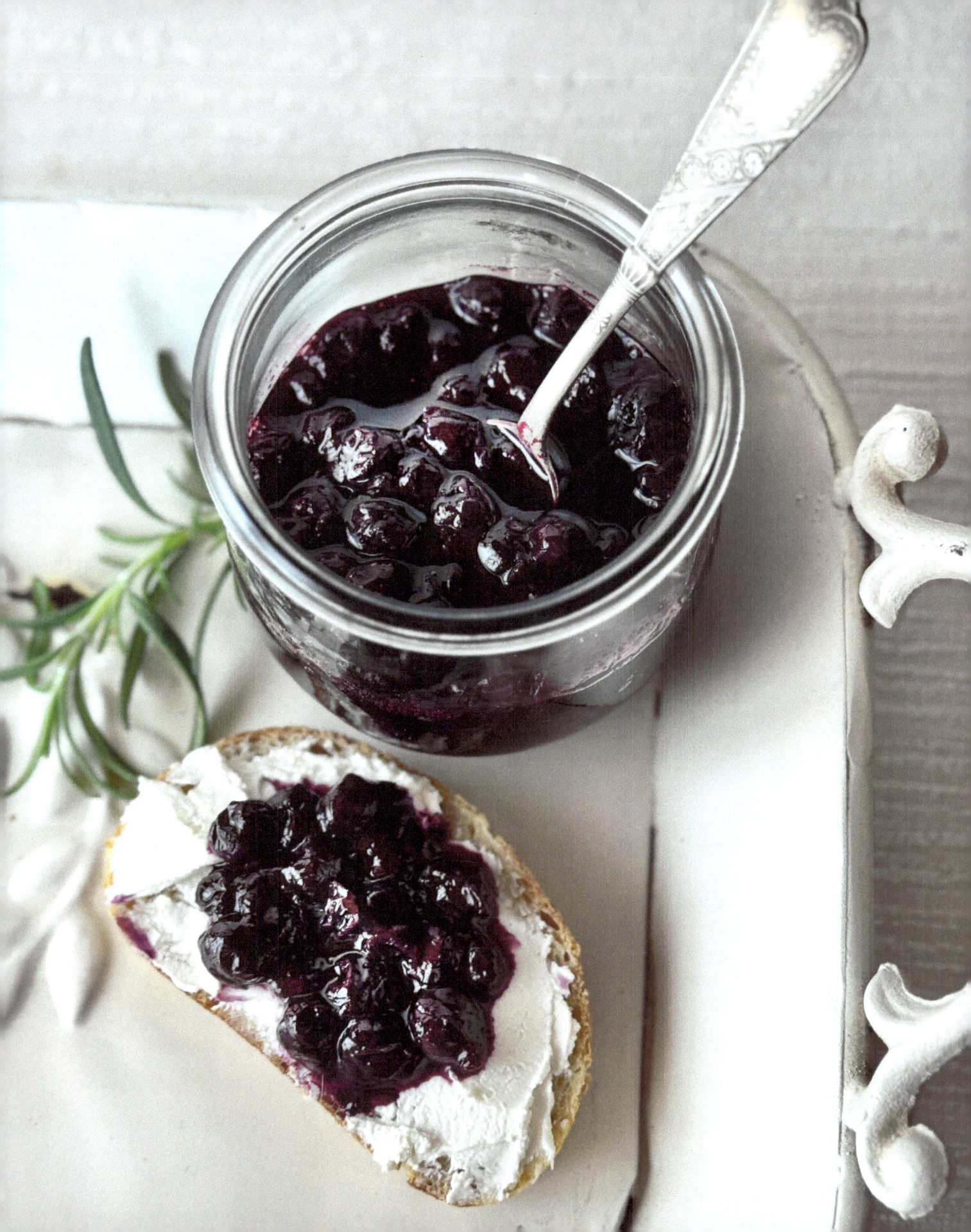

CONDIMENTS & PRESERVES

- Basic Blueberry Simple Syrup
- Pickled Blueberries
- Blueberry Salsa Macha
- Blueberry Bourbon BBQ Sauce
- Blueberry Corn Salsa
- Dried Blueberries
- Shrub Syrup
- Award-winning Blueberry Lavender Merlot Jam

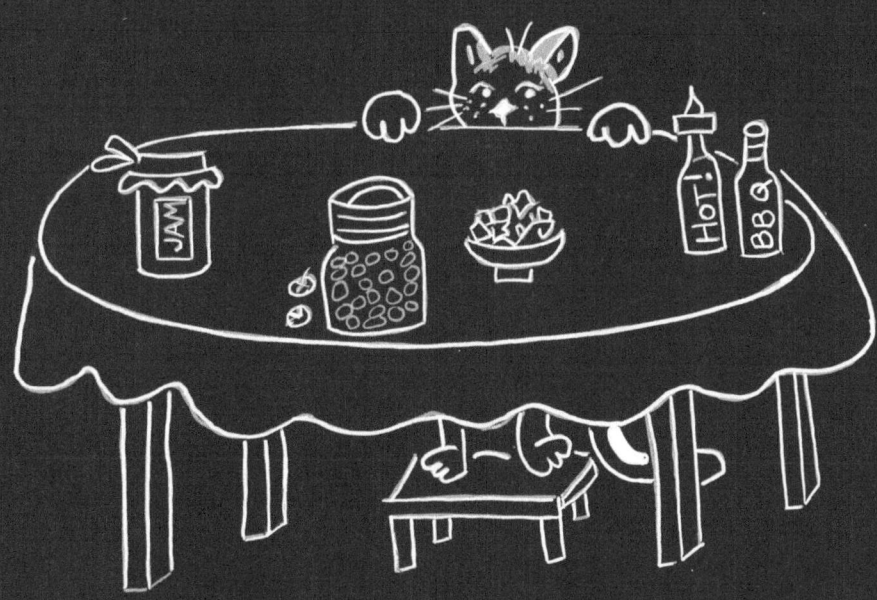

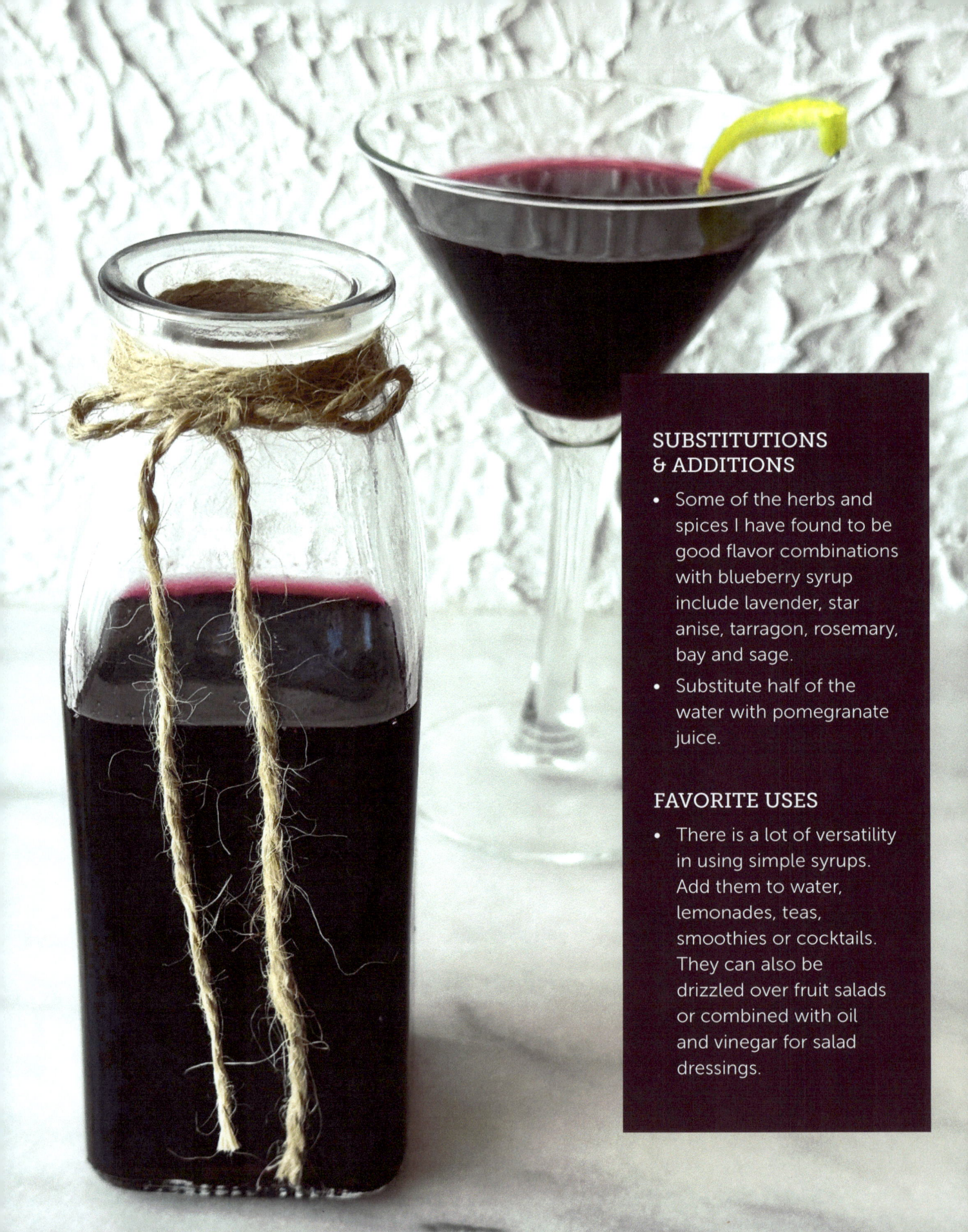

SUBSTITUTIONS & ADDITIONS

- Some of the herbs and spices I have found to be good flavor combinations with blueberry syrup include lavender, star anise, tarragon, rosemary, bay and sage.
- Substitute half of the water with pomegranate juice.

FAVORITE USES

- There is a lot of versatility in using simple syrups. Add them to water, lemonades, teas, smoothies or cocktails. They can also be drizzled over fruit salads or combined with oil and vinegar for salad dressings.

🥄 *EASY — Makes 1 ½ cup blueberry simple syrup (24 tablespoons)*

Basic Blueberry Simple Syrup

Italian sodas are essentially flavored syrups + carbonated water + fruit garnish. Add a little cream to the mix and you have a French Soda! The secret to a "great" Italian soda however is using real fruit, no corn syrup and herbal or spice infusions in your simple syrup.

• •

INGREDIENTS

For the Basic Simple Syrup Recipe:

  1 cup white granulated sugar

  1 cup water

  1 cup (8 oz) fresh blueberries

  1 teaspoon lemon juice

  ¼ cup herbs or ⅛ cup whole spices
  (i.e., allspice berries, pink peppercorns, etc.)

DIRECTIONS

1. To a small saucepan cook sugar and water over medium heat, stirring until sugar dissolves (about 2 minutes).
2. Add the blueberries, lemon juice and herbs or spices to the pan and stir together. Reduce heat to low and simmer for about 10 minutes, or until berries have burst.
3. Strain the berry mixture through a mesh sieve into a glass bottle with a lid or stainless steel covered container.
4. Syrups keep in the refrigerator for up to 1 month.

COOKING NOTES

- Mashing the berries while they are cooking can result in a cloudy syrup. Just let them simmer in the pot and cool before straining.

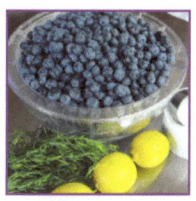

1. Gather ingredients

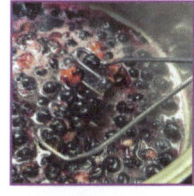

2. Cook and mash berries

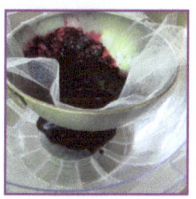

3. Strain berries

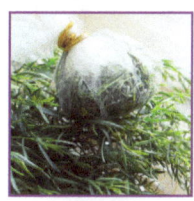

4. Add infusion and berries to pot and simmer

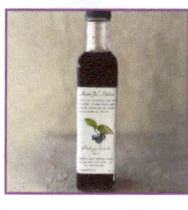

5. Pour into bottles

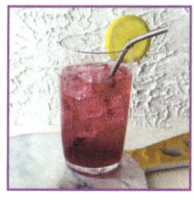

6. Craft your drink!

Nutrition Notes (per tablespoon): Calories 42; Protein 0.1g; Carbs 11g; Fat 0.1g; Sugar 10g

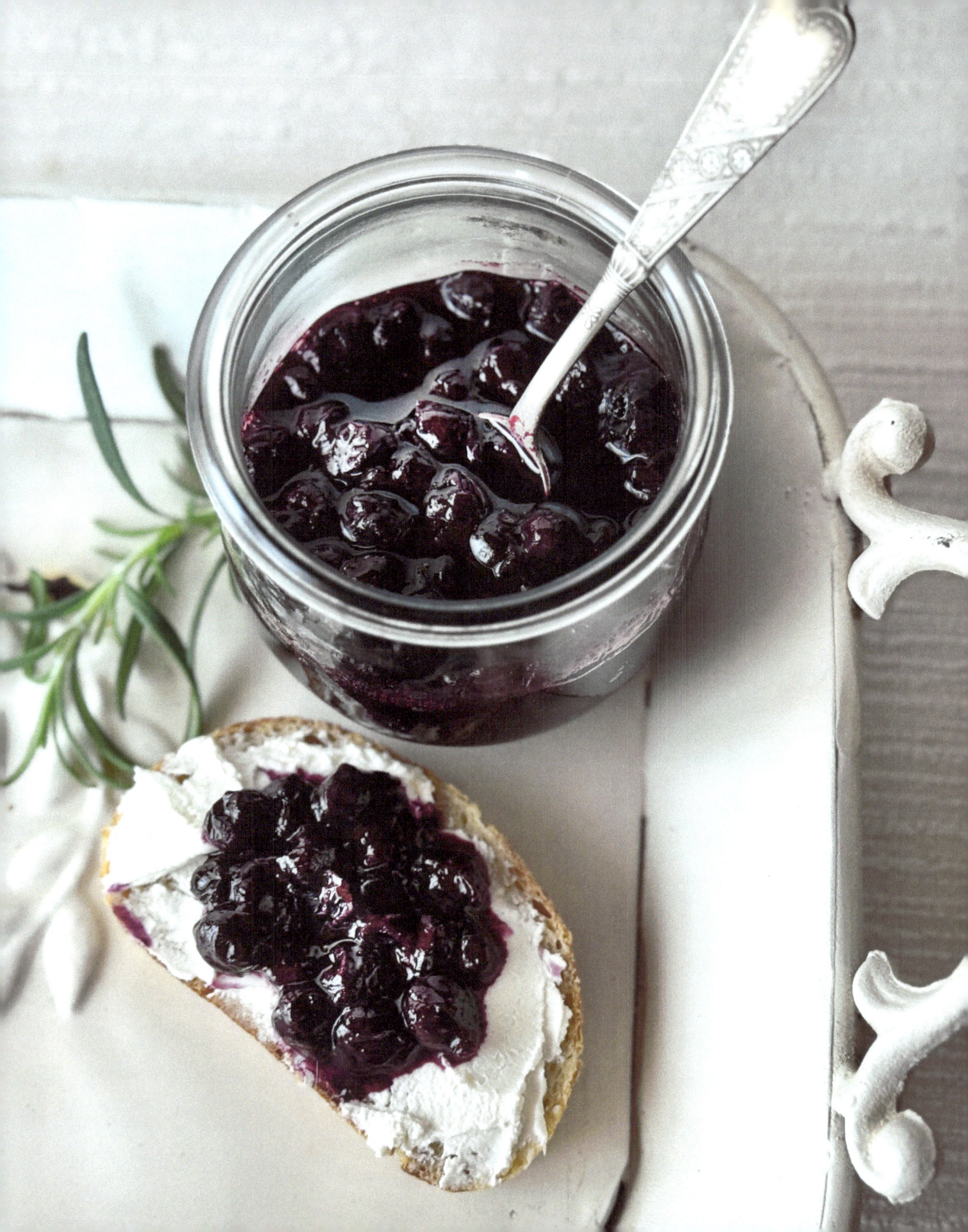

EASY — Makes a 12 oz (¾ to 1 pint) jar

Pickled Blueberries

This did not sound appealing to me at all—until I saw them being used with goat cheese on a charcuterie plate. That was a game changer, and now I always include these simple, unique pickled blueberries during any social gathering where a cheese platter might appear. They also make an excellent spread on ham sandwiches, or use them to make a flatbread pizza come alive (see the pizza recipe in the savory dinner section).

INGREDIENTS

1 cup (237 ml) white wine vinegar

1 cinnamon stick (5-inch)

6 whole cloves

2 whole allspice berries

2 whole star anise

½ cup (100 g) sugar

1 teaspoon kosher salt

2½ cups (15 oz) fresh or frozen blueberries

SUBSTITUTIONS & ADDITIONS

- Most vinegars can be substituted for white wine vinegar as long as they are at least 4% acidity. Rice wine vinegar is not recommended as it is typically less than 4%.
- Add strips of lemon peel to the jar for additional flavor. Ginger root or onions can be added but it will reduce storage time.

DIRECTIONS

1. Add vinegar and spices to a medium saucepan and bring to a low boil over medium heat. Reduce heat and simmer for 5 minutes. Remove pan from heat and let the spices sit in the vinegar to infuse for about 30 minutes.
2. With a slotted spoon, remove the whole spices and discard (or re-use in another batch). Add the sugar and salt to the pan and heat over medium heat, stirring until sugar dissolves (about 1 minute).
3. Add blueberries to the pan and bring to a low boil, stirring them in gently so as not to burst the berries. Allow the berries to boil without stirring any further for 5 minutes. Tip the pot back and forth occasionally to mix.
4. Remove from heat and use a slotted spoon to transfer the blueberries to a glass jar, along with enough pickling liquid to cover them.
5. Cover and refrigerate 24 hours before using to meld flavors. Pickled blueberries will keep covered and refrigerated for up to 3 months, but you should use within a couple of weeks for optimal flavor and texture.

Nutrition Notes (per teaspoon): Calories 10; Protein 0.04g; Carbs 2g; Fat 0.02g; Sugar 2g

MODERATE — Makes 2 cups Salsa Macha; Makes 1 cup Blueberry Salsa

Blueberry Salsa Macha

One of the most popular recipes on my food blog is for salsa macha. I use it with tortilla chips, over grilled chicken or fish, and as a topping for tacos or quesadillas. Adding a couple of teaspoons to a simple blueberry salsa resulted in a truly unique flavor profile that was both sweet and savory with a complex kick from the mixed peppers. The recipe below is actually three recipes—1 for the salsa macha, 1 for the blueberry salsa, and 1 for the delicious combination!

COOKING NOTES

- You can remove the seeds from the chile peppers, but it's not a must. Wear gloves when de-seeding hot peppers, especially for sensitive skin.
- It's important not to burn the garlic and chile peppers, as it will turn them bitter and ruin the flavor of your salsa macha.

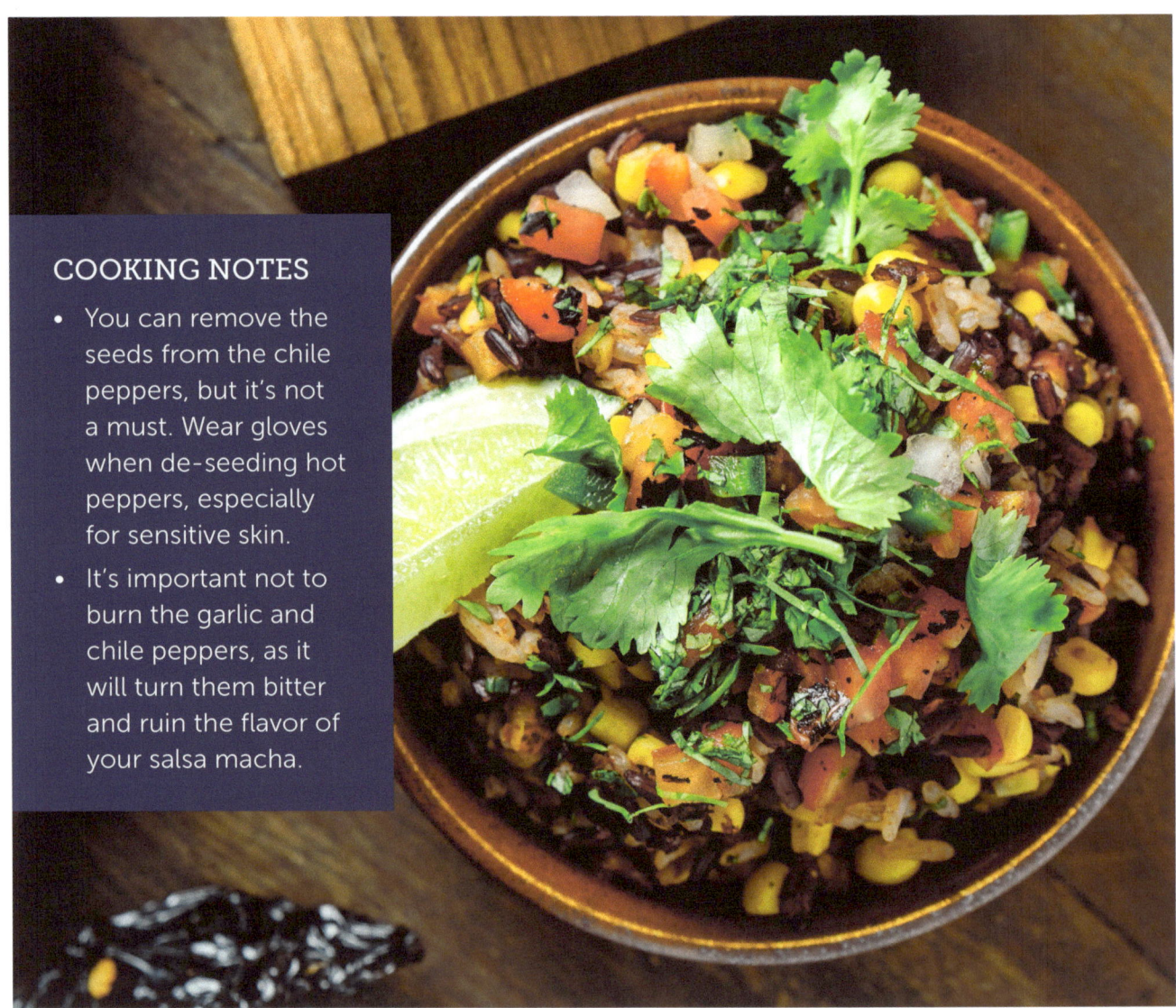

132 • THE BLUEBERRY COOKBOOK

INGREDIENTS

For the Salsa Macha / Chile Oil:

1 cup (236 ml) olive oil (see notes)

5 cloves garlic sliced

20 chiles de árbol stems removed

5 chiles moritas stems removed

½ cup (55 g) peanuts raw, unsalted

1 tablespoon sesame seeds

1 tablespoon vinegar whitecor apple cider

salt to taste

For the Blueberry Salsa:

1 cup (6 oz) fresh blueberries

¼ cup red onion, chopped

1 teaspoon lime zest

3 tablespoons (44 ml) fresh lime juice

3 tablespoons cilantro leaves

Salt and pepper to taste

DIRECTIONS

For the Salsa Macha / Chile Oil:

1. Heat the olive oil in the frying pan over medium to medium-low heat. It shouldn't be really hot or smoking. If you are using a cast iron skillet, know that it retains its heat once brought up to temp. It is easy to burn the ingredients so be careful of the temp and move quickly.

2. Toast the garlic slices until golden brown (about 30 seconds), and remove with a slotted spoon and set aside to cool off a bit.

3. Toast the chile peppers for about a minute in the same oil, until their color darkens (about 1 minute). Remove and set aside.

4. Toast the peanuts in the skillet until they reach golden brown (about 1 minute). Remove and set aside to cool. Reserve the oil in a small bowl.

5. Add the sesame seeds and the vinegar to the blender along with the cooled garlic, peppers, and peanuts. Pulse until the desired consistency is reached. Leave some bits, you don't want to turn your chili oil into chili paste!

6. Pour into a jar with a sealable lid and add the oil back in. Mix well and add salt to taste. Store in an airtight container in the refrigerator for up to 1 month. It will make about 2 cups and can be used in a number of different ways.

For the Fresh Blueberry Salsal:

Combine blueberries, onion, lime zest, lime juice, cilantro and salt and pepper in a food processor and pulse 5-6 times, until desired consistency.

For the Fresh Blueberry Salsa with Salsa Macha

Add 2-3 teaspoons of the homemade salsa macha (recipe above) to the blueberry salsa, mixing gently to incorporate the flavors and textures. Serve at room temperature with a side of lime wedges and more cilantro for those who like it. It will keep, covered, in the refrigerator for 3-7 days.

Nutrition For Salsa Macha Preserve (per teaspoon salsa macha):
Calories 20; Protein 1g; Carbs 2g; Fat 1g; Sugar 1g

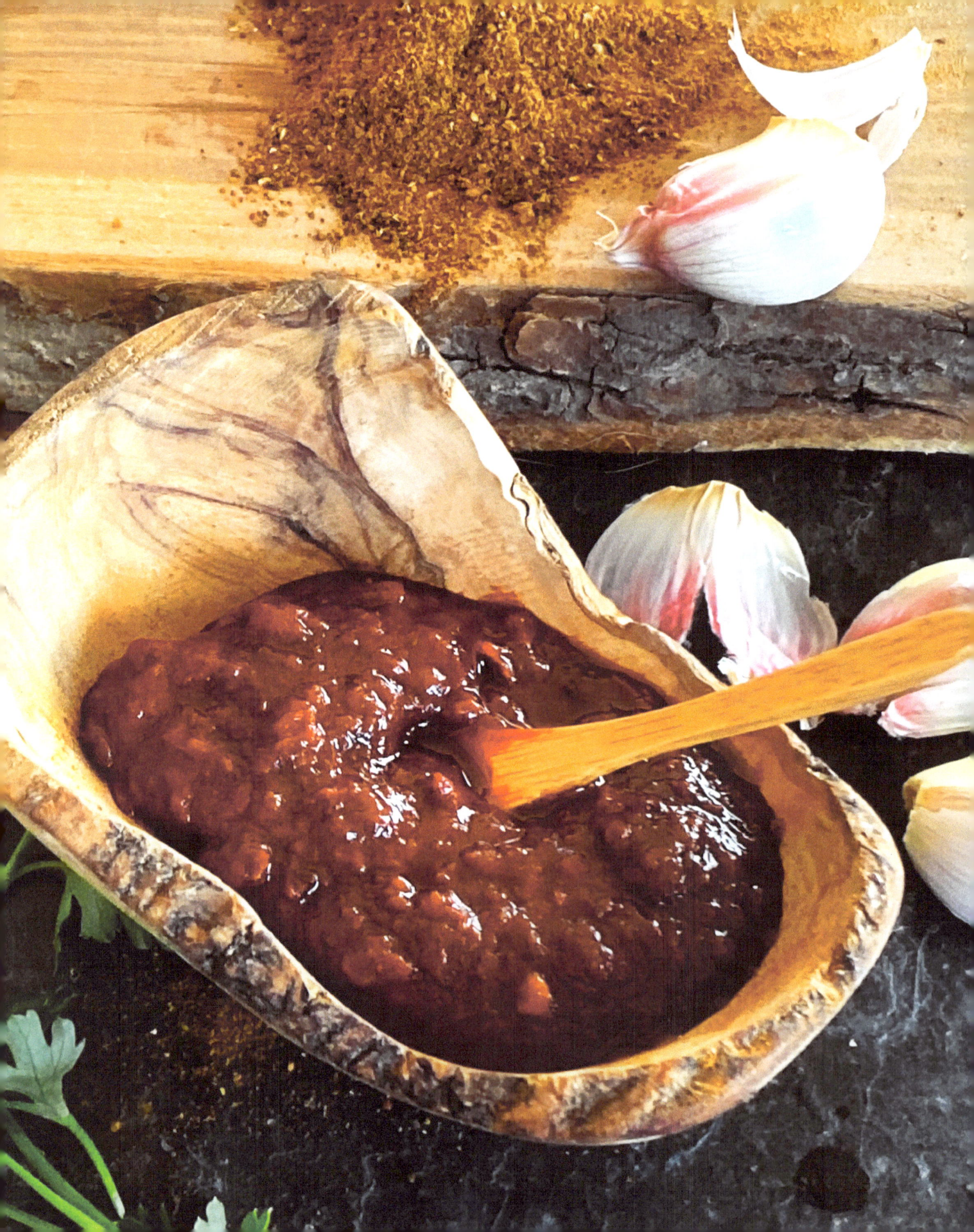

EASY — Makes 1 pint (32 tablespoons)

Blueberry Bourbon BBQ Sauce

This robust, savory BBQ sauce makes so many average dishes special, from a simple hamburger to Atlantic salmon to an expensive rib eye steak. I've even used it to level up a grilled cheese sandwich! I like mine with a bit of bourbon, but it is a stellar sauce sans alcohol.

INGREDIENTS

½ teaspoon hot sauce (I used Cholula)

½ teaspoon liquid smoke

½ cup (117 g) ketchup

¼ cup (59 ml) balsamic vinegar

3-4 tablespoons brown sugar (packed down)

3 tablespoons Dijon mustard

⅛ teaspoon ground allspice

1 tablespoon oil

½ medium onion, chopped

3 cloves garlic, minced

⅓ cup (79 ml) bourbon (optional)

3 cups (18 oz) blueberries (fresh or frozen)

½ teaspoon kosher salt

DIRECTIONS

1. Stir together the first 7 ingredients (hot sauce through allspice). Set aside.

2. Add 1 tablespoon oil to a large skillet and heat over medium heat. When hot, add the chopped onions and sauté for about 3-5 minutes or until caramelized. Add the garlic and cook for 30 seconds.

3. Add the bourbon (if using) and bring to a low boil for about 2 minutes. Add the blueberries, the salt and the reserved spice-vinegar mixture, stir and bring to a low boil. Reduce the heat to low and simmer for about 20 minutes, or until thickened to your preference.

4. Cool and refrigerate until ready to use, up to 2 weeks.

COOKING NOTES

- This sauce is quite robust and tangy so it pairs well with strong flavors (i.e., ribs, pork chops, etc.).
- Frozen blueberries work just fine with this recipe.
- This recipe boils the sauce first and then simmers it for 20 minutes, so most of the alcohol has evaporated. It does still have some residual alcohol, so feel free to leave it out.

Nutrition Notes (per tablespoon): Calories 23; Protein 0.2 g; Carbs 5 g; Fat 1 g; Sugar 4 g

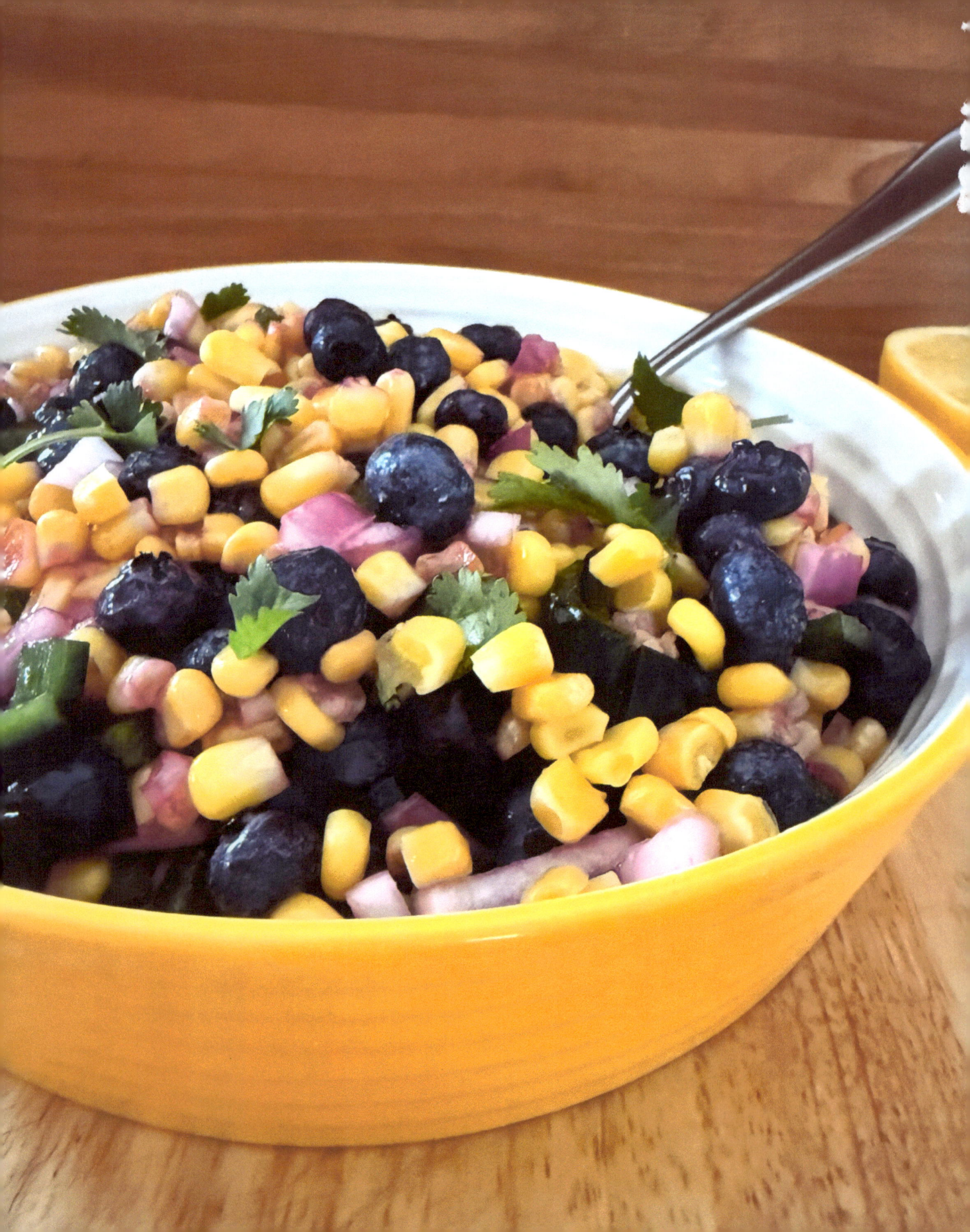

EASY — Makes 5 cups (10-12 servings)

Blueberry Corn Salsa

This salsa is the epitome of late summer to me. The end of the blueberry season in Minnesota lines up perfectly with the beginning of the fresh corn season and this salsa takes advantage of that timing. A favorite saying that I heard somewhere when I first started farming was "if it grows together, it goes together". I have found this to be true many times over, and it is especially true with blueberries and corn.

INGREDIENTS

4 tablespoons white wine vinegar

2 teaspoons lemon juice

6 tablespoons olive oil

2 cups (12 oz) fresh blueberries

3 cups (450 g) corn kernels, fresh or defrosted frozen

⅓ cup (50 g) diced purple onion

¼ cup (40 g) diced poblano pepper

½ teaspoon kosher salt

¼ cup cilantro or basil leaves

SUBSTITUTIONS & ADDITIONS

- If using frozen corn kernels, make sure the package doesn't contain a sauce. Allow them to dry thoroughly before using.
- Substitute your favorite chile pepper for the poblano pepper.
- You can use frozen blueberries in the salsa but it is best with fresh berries.

DIRECTIONS

1. In a small bowl whisk together the vinegar, lemon juice, and olive oil. Set aside and let the flavors meld together.
2. In a large bowl combine the blueberries, corn kernels, onion, poblano pepper and salt.
3. Add the herbs and the reserved dressing to the salsa and gently toss everything together.

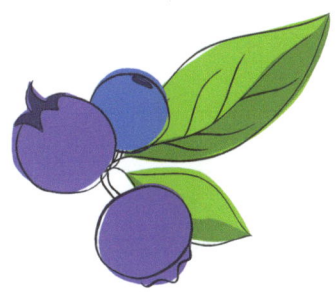

Nutrition Notes (per serving): Calories 113; Protein 2 g; Carbs 11 g; Fat 8 g; Sugar 5 g

MODERATE – 3 cups fresh berries = 1 ¼ cup dried; dehydrator recommended

Dried Blueberries

Dried fruit is very concentrated and some baked goods are actually preferable with dried blueberries over fresh. I find the raisin-like texture to excel in things like scones or oatmeal cookies (see recipes in this book). If you don't have a dehydrator, oven drying will work also, but the result is not as predictable and takes quite a long time.

The drying endpoint depends on your intended use. Drying to a raisin-like texture will work best for rehydrating to use in baked goods or as a snack within a short timeframe, but they will not keep forever without molding. Drying to the point of crispiness will allow an infinite shelf life, similar to the freeze dried blueberries you see in grocery stores.

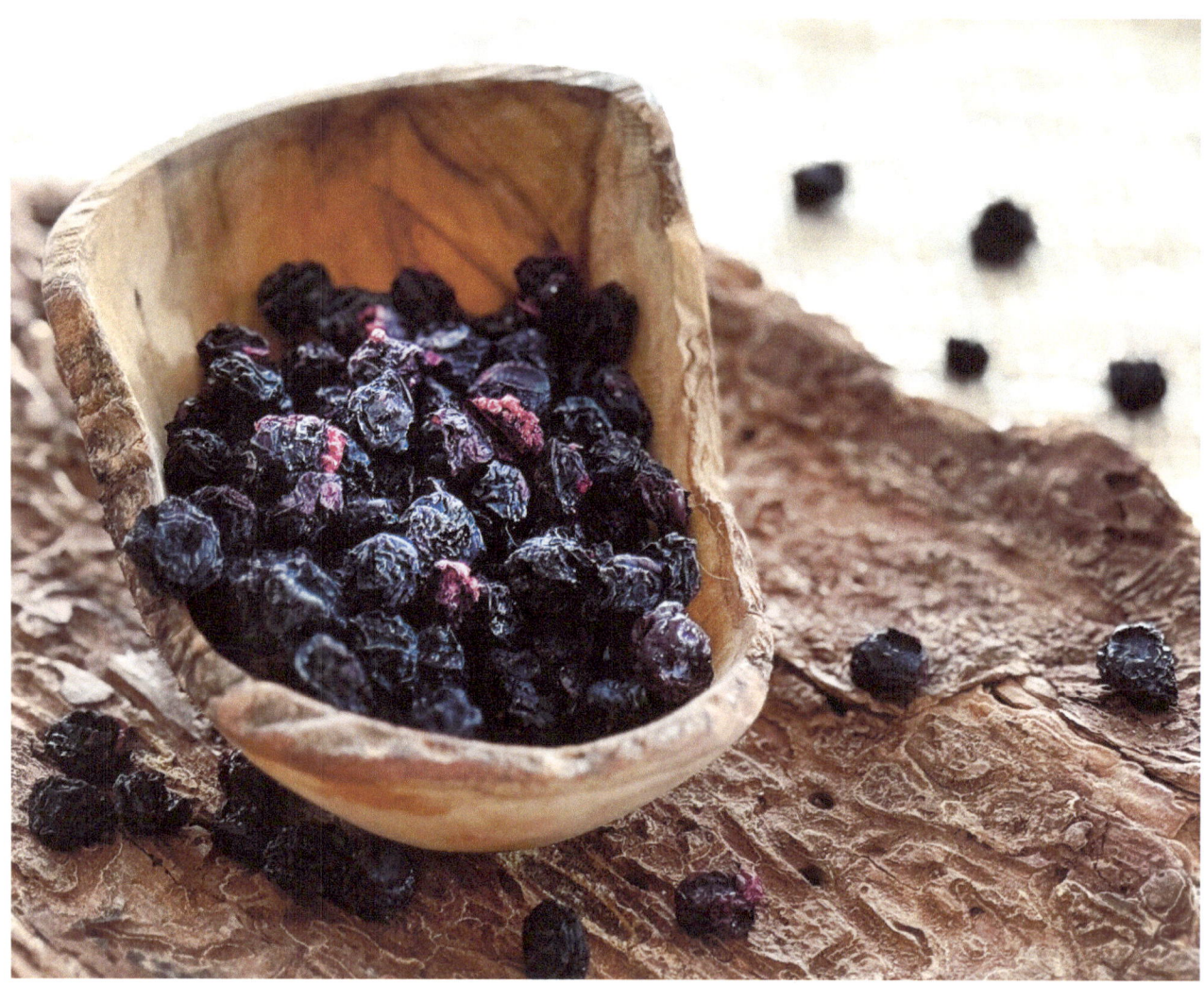

INGREDIENTS

3 cups (18 oz) blueberries (fresh or frozen)

DIRECTIONS

If your berries are fresh (preferred but not essential), blanch them first to get the best color, the most even texture, and the most flavor. If you are using frozen blueberries, pat them dry with paper towels and place on the racks in a single layer without blanching.

To Blanch Blueberries

Simply cover the berries with water in a saucepan and bring to a boil. While the berries are heating up to a boil, fill a large bowl with ice cubes and cold water. When the water in the saucepan comes to a boil, use a slotted spoon to remove the berries and add them to the ice water for about 30 seconds.

1. Remove the berries from the ice bath with the slotted spoon and place them on paper towels and pat them dry.

To Dry in a Dehydrator

Once berries are patted dry, place them on the dehydrator racks in a single layer, making sure to allow space between the berries. They should not be touching each other.

2. Turn the dehydrator on to 125° to 135°F (49-57°C). Allow the berries to dry for 18-24 hours or longer (depending on your dehydrator and how dry you want the texture). Check them every few hours to see if they are getting to the stage you prefer. I like mine to have the texture of raisins.

3. When they are at the stage you prefer, let them cool and then store them in an airtight container. The drier they are, the longer they will keep.

DRYING NOTES

- To speed up the dehydrating process, prick each blueberry with a toothpick.
- To dry in an oven, follow steps 1 through 4 and place them on a parchment-lined baking sheet in a 130°F (55°C) oven for about 10 hours.

STORAGE NOTES

- Because there are no preservatives added when drying fresh blueberries, they can mold if not dried thoroughly. Commercial raisins will last in a moist, chewy state because they have preservatives added.
- For optimal shelf life, store dried berries in a sealed container in a cool, dark pantry or cupboard..
- If you are going to use dried blueberries within 4 to 6 weeks, it will be fine to store them in a fairly chewy state. If you plan to keep them long term however, they need to be thoroughly dried. Perfectly dried blueberries can be stored for 6-12 months.

REHYDRATION NOTES

To rehydrate dried blueberries, just place them in a bowl of warm water to cover. Let them soak for about 30-60 minutes, depending on how soft you want them. Once they are rehydrated to your desired consistency, drain any excess water. The berries should then be plump.

Nutrition Notes (for 2oz): Calories 198; Protein 1g; Carbs 44g; Fat 1g; Sugar 30g

MODERATE – Makes 2 1/2 cups (40 tablespoons)

Shrub Syrup

Flavored vinegar fruit syrups added to carbonated water makes what is referred to as an old-fashioned "shrub". A shrub syrup (aka drinking vinegar) is essentially a concentrated fruit syrup with vinegar added. Sound weird? It was a very popular drink in the Colonial era when refrigeration wasn't available and vinegar could act as a preservative.

While the ingredients are simple, there is a debate on the best method for making shrub syrups. I generally use a hot shrubbing method as it is quicker, but some cooks or mixologists believe that a cold processing method results in a flavor that is more intense and pure. Both methods are included below.

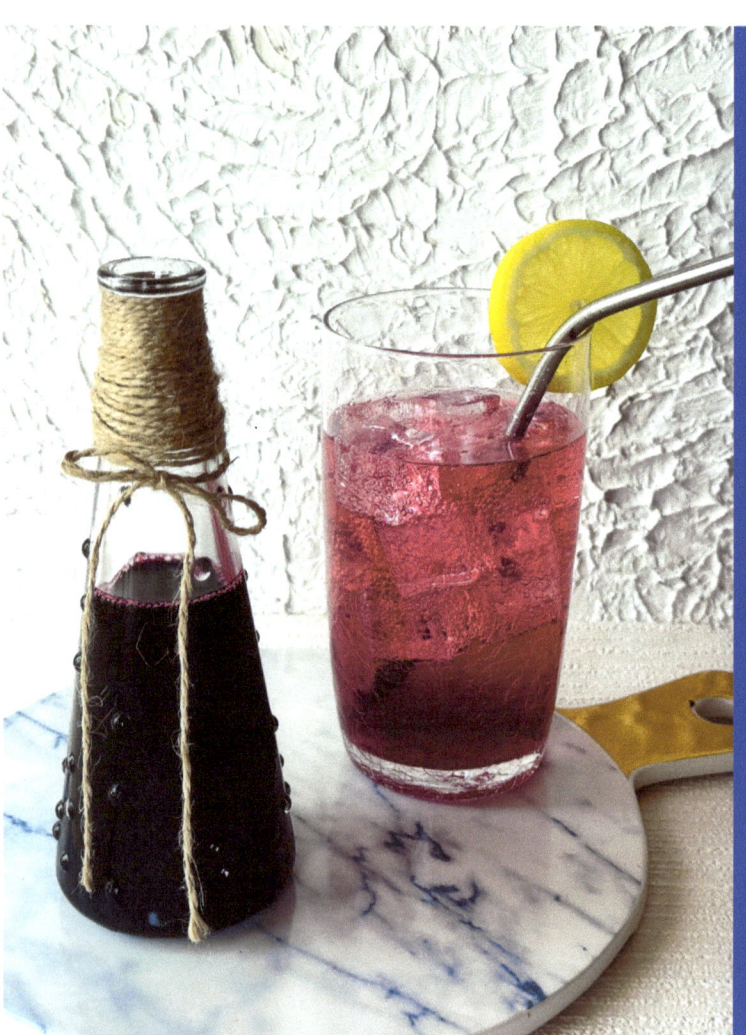

DID YOU KNOW

The American version of a shrub syrup originated in the 17th century, when vinegar was used to preserve berries and other fruits. This sweet and sour syrup of Colonial times was most often mixed with water and served as a refreshing drink while relaxing on the porch or to offer those working in the field.

INGREDIENTS

1 cup (6 oz) blueberries (fresh or thawed frozen)

1 cup (200 g) granulated sugar

1 cup (237 ml) apple cider vinegar

ADDING HERBAL/SPICE INFUSIONS

- Adding herbal or spice infusions to shrub syrups is a fun way to customize and add flavor. For blueberry shrub syrups I've successfully tried infusions of lavender, tarragon, pink peppercorns and pomegranate.
- To make an infusion, place your preferred herbs or spices in a square of cheesecloth, gather it into a pouch, and secure it with a rubber band or a tie.
- For cold processing, just drop the infusion bag into the container, making sure it is covered by the liquid. Remove the bag when your shrub syrup is ready.
- For hot processing, add the infusion bag to the pot after the sugar has dissolved and after you have added the vinegar. Bring the mixture to a boil and then turn off the heat and let the infusion bag steep into the syrup for 20-30 minutes. Then remove the bag and pour the syrup into bottles.
- Shrub syrups will keep for several months, as both vinegar and sugar are preservatives.

DIRECTIONS

Cold Shrubbing Process for Blueberry Shrub Syrup:

1. Stir the berries and sugar together in a stainless steel bowl or large pickle jar and allow them to steep 6-12 hours to release their juices.
2. Strain the berry-sugar mixture through a fine mesh into a glass or stainless steel container to remove the pulp or solids (try and let them drain without mashing them too much to avoid a cloudy syrup).
3. Add the vinegar to the container and stir to combine.
4. Cover the container with a lid and allow it to sit undisturbed for 15-30 days.
5. Pour into bottles and refrigerate until ready to use.

Hot Shrubbing Process for Blueberry Shrub Syrup:

1. This method is quick and easy if you have some sort of juicer. Because it comes to a rolling boil, it will be pasteurized and will therefore be shelf stable. Flavors will mellow after a couple of months.
2. Juice the blueberries and discard the pulp (or use pulp elsewhere). I use a commercial steam juicer called a Mehu Liisa to extract the juice. It is basically a double boiler where you add fruit to a large colander type of pot that steams the fresh fruit into juice collected in a middle pot that releases the juice to a container through gravity-fed tubing (see photo). Of course, you can use a regular juicer also.
3. Add the blueberry juice and sugar to a large pot and heat over medium-high until the sugar is dissolved (about 2 minutes). Stir the vinegar into the pot.
4. Bring the syrup-vinegar mixture up to a rolling boil to pasteurize and then pour into hot bottles.

Nutrition Notes (per tablespoon): Calories 23; Protein .03g; Carbs 6g; Fat .03g; Sugar 5g

🥄🥄🥄 DIFFICULT — Yield: 9 8-oz jars (half-pints)

Blueberry Lavender Merlot Jam

This low sugar jam was a national award winner (Good Food Awards - 2013) and was the impetus for developing a wide range of farm-fresh jams, jellies, syrups and sauces from our farm. We built a commercial kitchen on the farm and sold our products online and at the Twin Cities farmers markets for 15 years. I've wound down the jam business but often make this particular recipe for myself or for gifts. It was always a market favorite and I love that it is low sugar and can be used for savory dishes also.

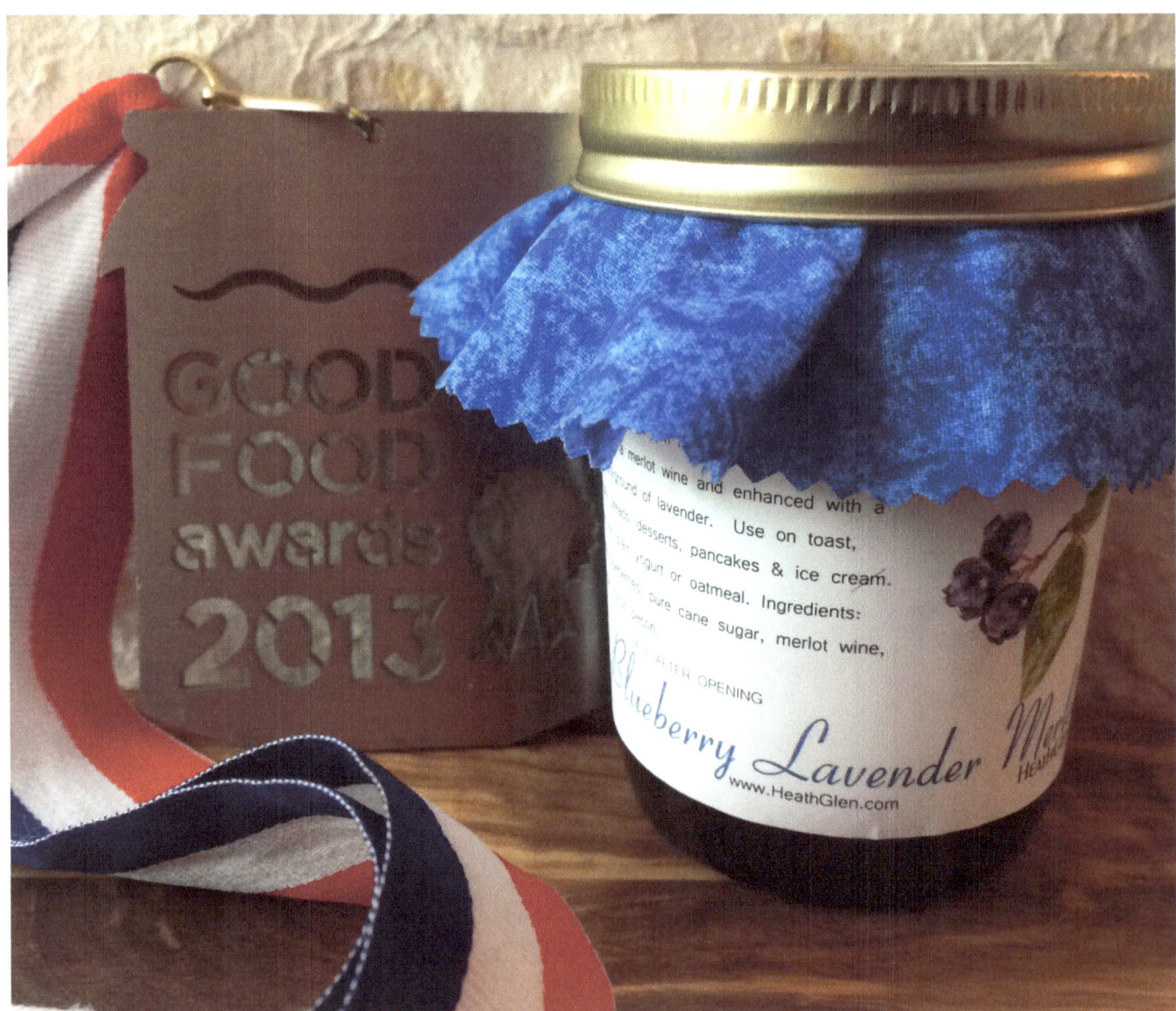

INGREDIENTS

6½ cups (39 oz) blueberries

2 tablespoons fresh lemon juice

1 cup (237 ml) merlot wine

½ cup culinary lavender

½ cup + 2 tablespoons L-M-3 Pacific Pectin (see notes)

4 cups (800 g) sugar

¼ teaspoon butter

COOKING NOTES

- More fruit is used for the amount of sugar, so the flavor is less sweet and allows the fruit to shine.
- I used a commercial low sugar pectin called L-M-3 by Pacific Pectin, a low-methoxyl pectin derived from citrus fruits. Other low sugar pectins on the market include Sure Jell Light, Ball 100% Natural Reduced Calorie Fruit pectin, Kerr Pure Fruit Pectin (lite), Slim Set Pectin, or Pomona Pectin. You will need to follow specific directions on those pectins, as all are a little different.
- Crystals in the jam can be a sign that the mixture was cooked too long or too slowly. Long slow cooking results in too much evaporation of water which will sometimes result in crystallization.

DIRECTIONS

1. Turn the oven on to 200°F. Place the half-pint jars in an oven-safe pan and place in the oven while making the jam.
2. Add the blueberries, lemon juice and wine to a large stainless steel pot and heat over medium heat. Use a potato masher to mash the berries a little as the mixture heats.
3. Add the lavender and turn the heat up to medium-high. Use a digital thermometer and when the mixture is heated to 130-140°F (54-60°C), stir in the low sugar pectin, and boil for 30 seconds to hydrate.
4. Add the sugar and quickly bring to a rolling boil (a boil that cannot be stirred down) and keep at rolling boil for 30 seconds to 1 minute, stirring constantly. Stir in butter to help reduce foaming.
5. Remove jars from the oven and pour jam into heated jars and secure with clean, unused lids and rings.
6. At this point you can sterilize the jam in the jars in a hot water bath for 5-10 minutes to increase shelf life or you can leave jars to cool on the countertop and seal naturally as they cool. The hot water bath will form a tighter seal and ensure that the jam is shelf stable. As long as you use hot jars and hot unused lids, the countertop method will work, but it will not seal as tightly so you need to test the lids after they have cooled. Many home cooks are comfortable with allowing the jars to seal on their own, but safety guidelines require water baths for long term storage.

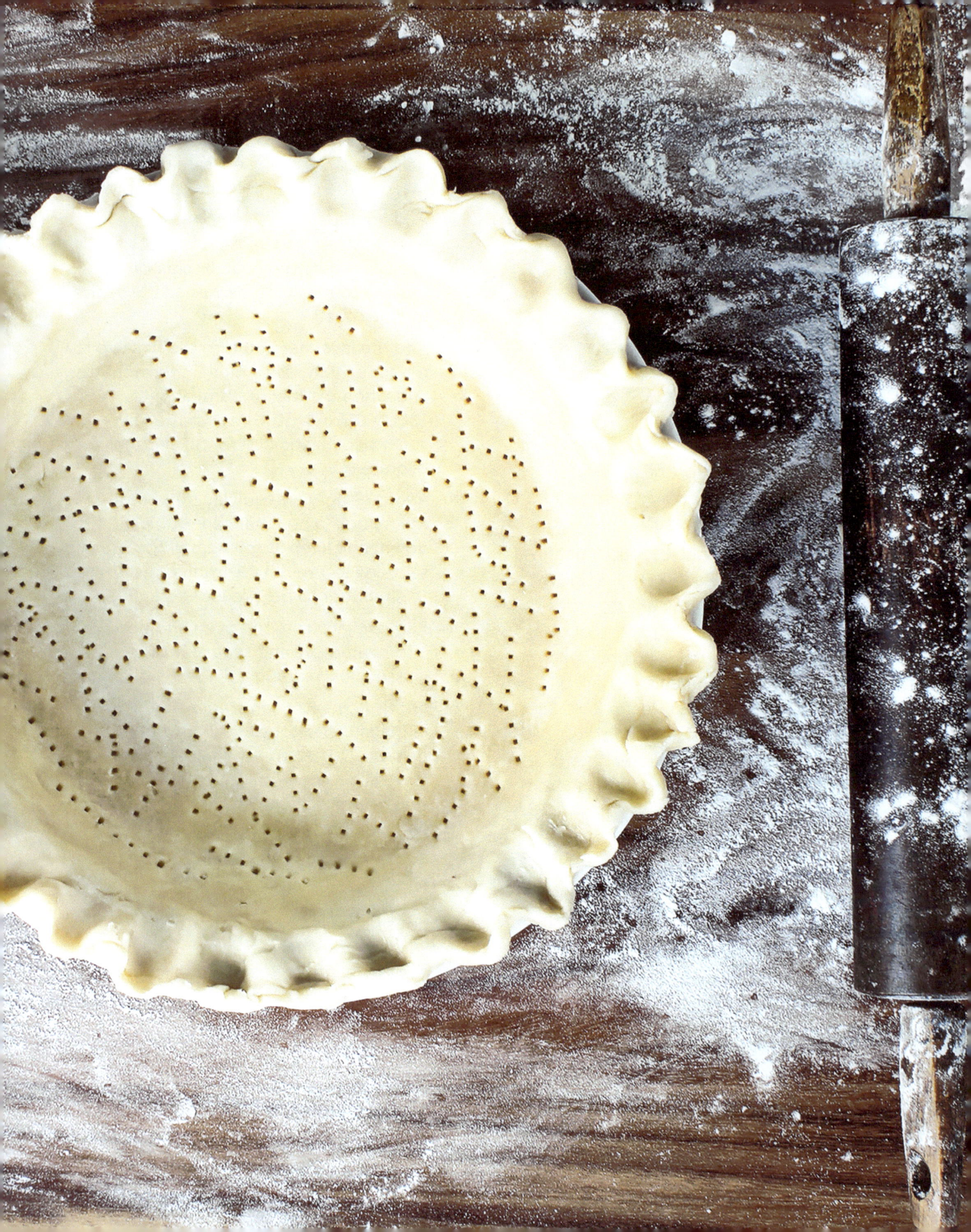

FOUNDATIONAL RECIPES

Crusts

Frostings

Sauces

Toppings

Vinegars/Vinaigrette

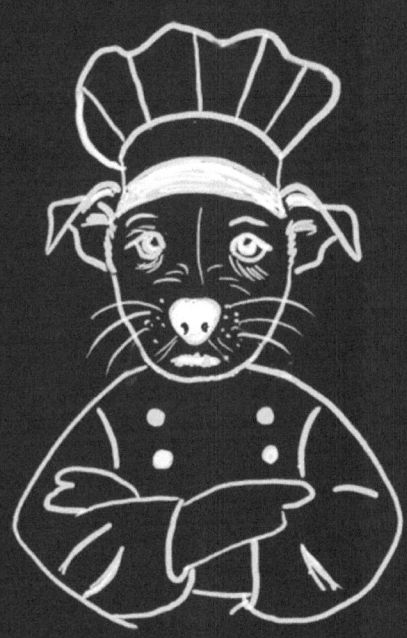

Crusts

CORNMEAL PIE CRUST

Makes 1 pie shell and lid (8-10 servings)
Chill time required — 1 hour +

Ingredients

2 ½ cups (300 g) all-purpose flour

¼ cup (37 g) cornmeal

3 tablespoons sugar

½ teaspoon salt

12 tablespoons (168 g) unsalted butter, chilled

¼ cup (50 g) vegetable shortening (or lard), chilled

4 tablespoons (60 ml) ice water

Directions

1. Fill a small bowl with ice water. In a food processor pulse together the flour, cornmeal, sugar and salt. Cut the butter and shortening into chunks over the processor bowl and pulse until you get a coarse meal texture. Add the ice water and pulse just enough to bring the dough together.

2. Empty the dough onto the counter and form into a ball (dough will be thick). Divide the dough into two even balls and flatten each into a disc. Do not knead the dough—work it as little as possible. Wrap each disc in plastic wrap and chill for at least 1 hour or up to 1 day ahead.

3. When ready to make the pie, remove the dough and filling from the refrigerator and let them sit for about 10-15 minutes to reach room temperature. While the dough is warming up, preheat the oven to 400°F (204°C) and grease your pie plate with butter or cooking spray.

4. Place the first dough disc between 2 pieces of parchment paper and roll out to a 12" round. Peel off the top piece of parchment paper and invert the dough round onto the pie plate, leaving a generous overhang. Peel off the top parchment paper and gently press the dough into the plate (if it cracks, just wet your fingers and smooth it back together). Add the blueberry filling to the pie.

5. Repeat the rollout process with the second dough disc and place it over the top of the filling, centering as much as possible. Peel off the top piece of parchment paper and crimp the dough together around the perimeter of the pie. You can get fancy and flute the edges or just push the top dough together with the bottom overhang to form a simple crust. Use a sharp knife and make five 2-3" slits on the top.

6. Brush the middle of the dough (not the edges) with a little milk or cream and sprinkle with sugar (turbinado sugar if you have it). Use the cream and sugar to mask any cracks in the top dough layer. Bake for 15 minutes and then reduce heat to 350°F (177°C) without opening the oven door. Continue baking for about 1 hour and 15 minutes, or until the crust is golden brown and the filling is bubbling through the slits in the crust. Look for the bubbling juices

so you don't underbake the pie, or it will be soupy.

7. If the crust along the rim starts to get too dark you can cover the edges of the crust with a little aluminum foil.

8. Cool on a rack for at least 4 hours for the filling to set.

GALETTE / CROSTATA (FREE-FORM PIE)

Makes one 12-14-inch crust
Chill time required — 1 hour or up to 3 days

Ingredients

1 ¼ cups (156 g) all-purpose flour

¼ cup (30 g) fine cornmeal

1 tablespoon granulated sugar

½ teaspoon salt

½ cup (113 g) unsalted butter, chilled

¼ cup (60 ml) buttermilk, cold (see substitutions below)

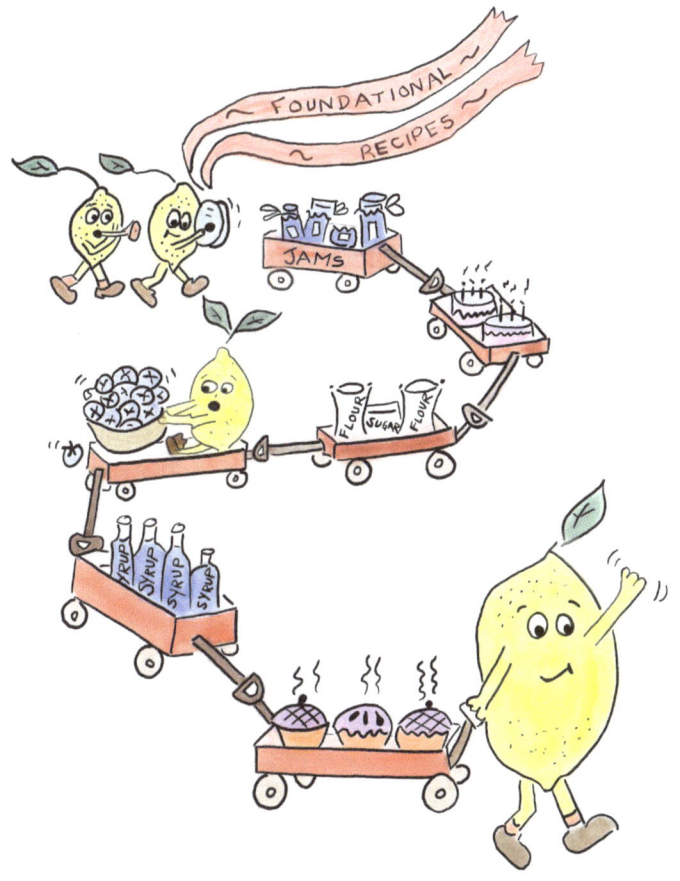

Directions

1. In a medium-sized bowl, whisk together the flour, cornmeal, sugar and salt. Working quickly, cut the chilled butter into chunks (½-inch cubes) and add to the bowl. Using a pastry cutter or a couple of forks or your hands, cut in the butter until the mixture is in pea-sized crumbs.

2. Stir in the buttermilk, adding another tablespoon if the dough seems dry.

3. Using your hands, bring the dough together into a ball and place on a lightly floured counter or surface and flatten it into a 1-inch thick disc. Do not handle the dough too much or it will get warm and overdeveloped. Wrap the disc of dough in plastic wrap and chill in the refrigerator for at least 1 hour or up to 3 days.

4. When you are ready to make the galette (aka crostata), preheat the oven to 425°F

(218°C) and line a rimmed baking sheet with parchment paper or a silicone mat. Leave the dough in the refrigerator while you make the filling.

5. Remove the chilled dough from the refrigerator, place on a lightly floured surface, and begin to roll out the dough to an approximate 12-14-inch circle. This is a freeform tart, so do not worry about the shape. I find it easier to roll up the edges if the shape is circular, but oblong can work also. Drape the dough over the rolling pin and transfer to the baking sheet lined with a silicone mat or parchment paper. It can overhang the baking sheet a bit.

6. Spread the filling onto the dough, leaving a 2-inch border around the edge. Don't pile the filling too high as it will be harder for the crust to bake all the way through and it may turn out mushy.

7. Working with 3-4 inches of length at a time, fold the edge of the dough up over the berry filling, pressing the seams together where they overlap. Repeat until all the edges are folded up. If the dough tears, wet your fingers and rub the dough to patch it up.

8. Place the galette in the freezer for 10-15 minutes, or until the dough is firm.

9. Remove the galette from the freezer and brush the edges of the dough with an egg wash (1 egg and 1-2 tablespoons milk or cream whisked together), and sprinkle with coarse sugar.

10. Bake for 20-25 minutes, or until the crust is golden brown and the filling is bubbling. The crust of a crostata is fairly thin and will burn quicker than a pie crust. Since all ovens are a bit different, check on your crostata during the bake time and remove when the crust is golden brown. It should take 20-25 minutes at 425°F (218°C), but some ovens will require a longer time. Cool for 10 minutes before serving.

Substitutions

If you don't have buttermilk handy, you can make this DIY mixture: In a liquid measuring cup add ½ teaspoon of fresh lemon juice or white vinegar and enough whole milk until it reaches ¼ cup. Stir and let it sit for 5 minutes before using it in the recipe.

Cooking Notes

For a galette, the dough needs to be a little stronger than for a pie to prevent the filling juices from oozing out around the galette and burning. This means that a galette dough needs to incorporate the butter into the flour more than a regular pie dough. The result is less flaky than a pie dough, but much more sturdy.

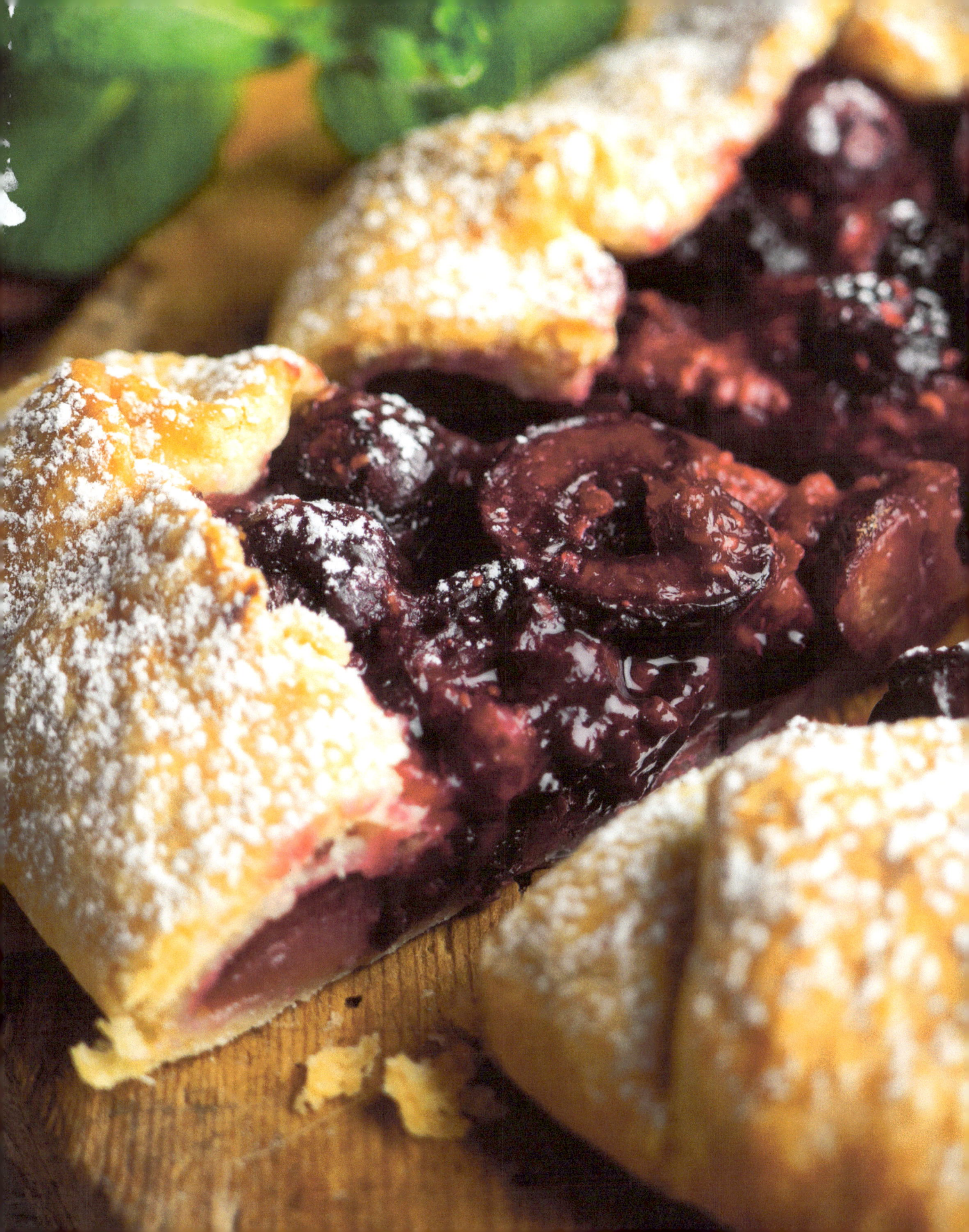

Frostings

BLUEBERRY BUTTERCREAM

Makes about 4 cups
Used with Lemon Ricotta Cookies

Ingredients

¾ cup (170 g) unsalted butter, softened to room temp.

3 ½ - 4 cups (420-480 g) powdered sugar

½ cup (130 g) blueberry jam or jelly

⅛ teaspoon salt

1 ½ teaspoons vanilla extract

2-3 tablespoons heavy cream (optional, if needed to thin frosting)

Directions

1. In a stand mixer or electric mixer, beat the softened butter on medium speed for 1-2 minutes, or until creamy.

2. On low speed add 1 cup of the powdered sugar slowly so it doesn't fly out of the bowl. Beat in the jelly, salt and vanilla and add the rest of the powdered sugar a little at a time.

3. If the frosting is too thick for your preference, add a little cream. If it is too thin, add more powdered sugar.

4. When the frosting is to your preferred thickness and smoothness, cover and refrigerate until ready to use. The frosting can be stored in the refrigerator for up to a week, or in the freezer for up to three months. The frosting may need to be re-whipped to restore its fluffy texture after chilling.

Cooking Notes

- To ensure success, have all your ingredients at room temperature, but especially the butter. Cold butter will not emulsify and the result will be a clumpy frosting.
- Room temperature butter is soft but not melted. Best practice is to just let it sit out on the counter for 1-2 hours.

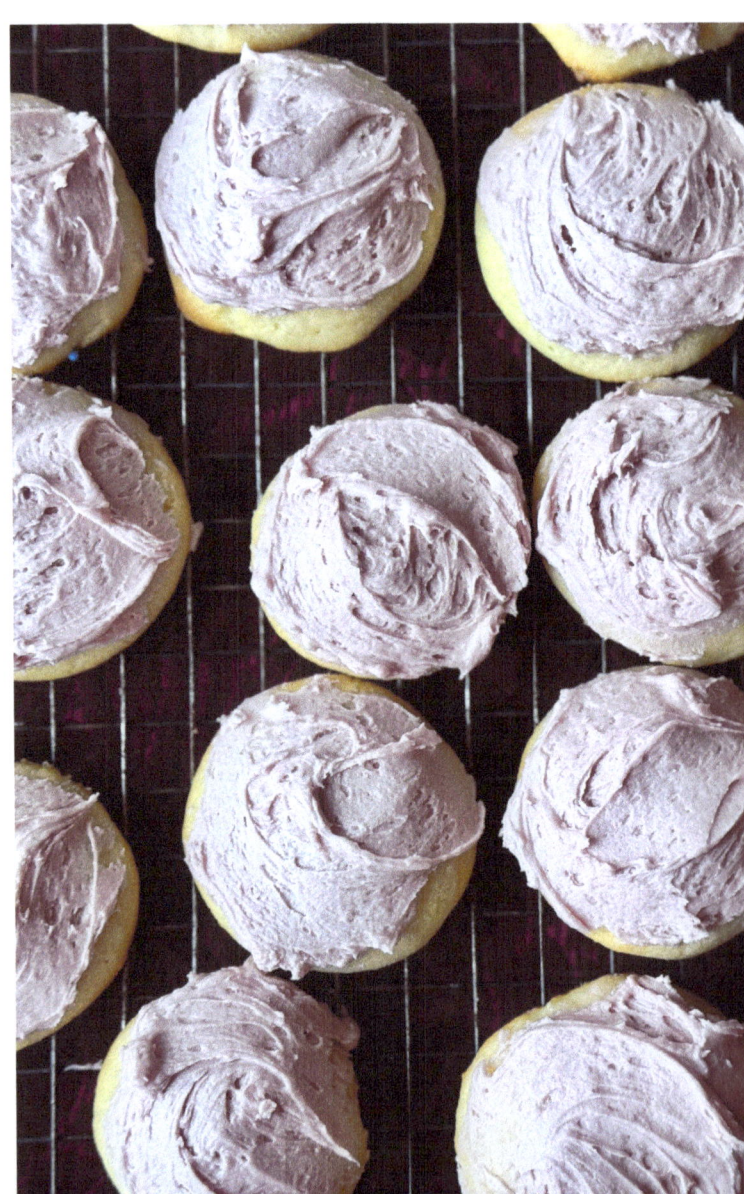

BLUEBERRY CREAM CHEESE FROSTING

Makes 4-5 cups
Used with Chocolate Sheet Cake

Ingredients

2 cups (12 oz) blueberries (I used frozen)

3 tablespoons sugar

1 tablespoon cornstarch

1 tablespoon lemon zest (grated zest from 1 medium lemon)

8 oz (226 g) full fat brick cream cheese (not a cream cheese spread), room temp.

½ cup (113 g) unsalted butter, room temp.

3 ¼ cups (375 g) powdered sugar

1 teaspoon vanilla

¼ teaspoon kosher salt

Directions

1. First make a blueberry compote by combining blueberries, sugar, cornstarch and lemon zest in a saucepan and cooking over medium heat until the compote thickens (about 3-5 minutes). Remove from heat and set aside to cool.

2. While the compote is cooling, beat together the cream cheese and butter in a handheld or stand mixer on high speed. It should look creamy and smooth.

3. Add the powdered sugar, vanilla and salt and beat for 2 more minutes (slowly at first until powdered sugar is a little incorporated), scraping the sides as you go. If you prefer a thicker frosting, add a little more powdered sugar. Cover and refrigerate.

4. When using the frosting on a cake, everything should be cool (the cake, the compote and the cream cheese frosting). Dollop spoonfuls of cream cheese frosting on the top of the cake and spread it around with a butter knife. Then drop spoonfuls of compote onto the cream cheese frosting and swirl the compote into the cream cheese frosting with a clean butter knife.

Cooking Notes

- It is sometimes easier to frost cakes if they are frozen, but make sure and wrap the cake tightly in plastic wrap if you freeze it so it won't dry out. Bring the frosting to room temperature so that you can easily spread it over the frozen cake adding swirls.

- You may have some compote left over. Just keep it in the refrigerator covered and use it on other baked goods.

- Any leftover cream cheese frosting will keep in the refrigerator for 5+ days or it can be frozen for up to 3 months.

Sauces

ALL-AROUND BLUEBERRY COMPOTE (SAUCE)

Makes 1 ¾ cups (about 12 servings)

Can be used in ice cream sandwiches, pancakes, sheet cake, crepes, and poke cake recipes.

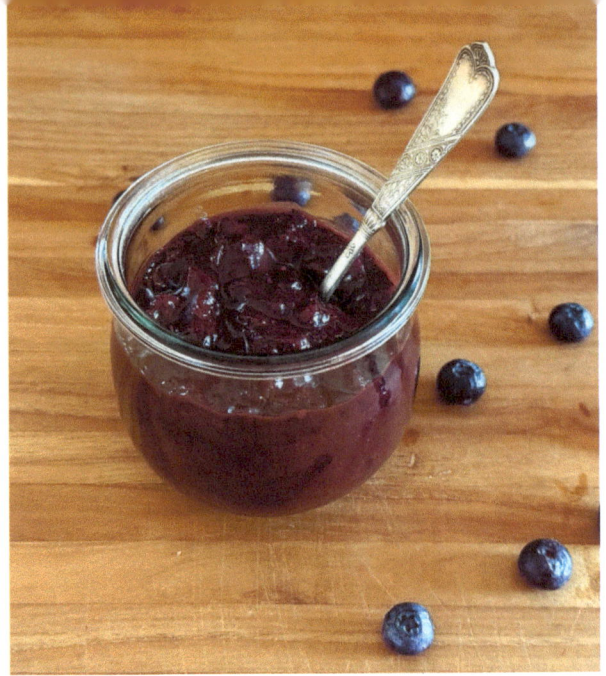

Ingredients

1 tablespoon lemon zest

2 tablespoons fresh lemon juice

2 cups (12 oz) fresh or frozen blueberries

¼ cup (50 g) granulated sugar

½ teaspoon vanilla

⅛ teaspoon salt

1 tablespoon cornstarch

1 tablespoon water

Directions

1. Zest a large lemon and set aside the zest. Cut the lemon in half and juice it to get about 2 tablespoons of juice.
2. In a small saucepan, whisk together the blueberries, sugar, lemon juice, lemon zest, vanilla and salt and bring to a boil over medium heat.
3. In a small bowl whisk together the cornstarch and water until no lumps remain. Add the cornstarch slurry to the saucepan and cook for 3-5 minutes, stirring often and mashing blueberries with a potato masher as it cooks.
4. When thickened to your preference, remove from heat and let it cool. The longer you cook it the thicker it will become.
5. For storage, cool completely and transfer to an airtight container and refrigerate for 1-2 weeks. Compote can be frozen in an airtight container or freezer-safe bag for up to 3 months.

Cooking Notes

The term "compote" is often interchanged with the terms sauce or coulis. The differences are subtle and not altogether relevant, but here is a breakdown:

- A compote is thicker than a sauce and will usually include whole berries. It is perfect for topping sheet cakes or ice cream;
- A fruit sauce is thinner and less chunky than a compote and might be used over pancakes or some of the savory meat dishes in this book;
- A coulis is pureed and then passed through a sieve, resulting in a more elegant dessert sauce to serve over crepes or pastries.

Nutrition Notes (per serving): Calories 33; Protein 0.2 g; Carbs 8 g; Fat 0.1 g; Sugar 7 g

BLUEBERRY BBQ SAUCE

Makes 2 cups
Used in savory main dishes
(ribs, pork chops and cheeseburger).

Ingredients

½ teaspoon hot sauce (I use Cholula)

½ teaspoon liquid smoke

½ cup (117 g) ketchup

¼ cup (59 ml) balsamic vinegar

3-4 tablespoons brown sugar (packed)

3 tablespoons Dijon mustard

⅛ teaspoon ground allspice

1 tablespoon oil

½ medium onion, chopped

3 cloves garlic, minced

⅓ cup (79 ml) bourbon (optional)

3 cups (18 oz) blueberries (fresh or frozen)

½ teaspoon kosher salt

Directions

1. In a bowl, stir together the first 7 ingredients (hot sauce through allspice). Set aside.
2. Add 1 tablespoon of oil to a large skillet and heat over medium heat. When hot add the chopped onions and sauté for about 3-5 minutes or until slightly caramelized. Add the garlic and cook for 30 seconds.
3. Add the bourbon (if using) and bring to a low boil for about 2 minutes. Add the blueberries, the salt and the reserved spice-vinegar mixture, stir and bring to a low boil. Reduce the heat to low and simmer for about 20 minutes, or until thickened to your preference.
4. Cool and refrigerate until ready to use, up to 2 weeks. If you want to make this shelf stable, you can run it through a water bath in the same way you would for canning a jelly.

Cooking Notes

- This sauce is quite robust and tangy so it pairs well with strong flavors (i.e., ribs, pork chops, etc.).
- Frozen blueberries work just fine with this recipe.
- This recipe boils the sauce first and then simmers it for another 20 minutes, so most of the alcohol has evaporated. It does still have some residual alcohol, so feel free to leave it out.

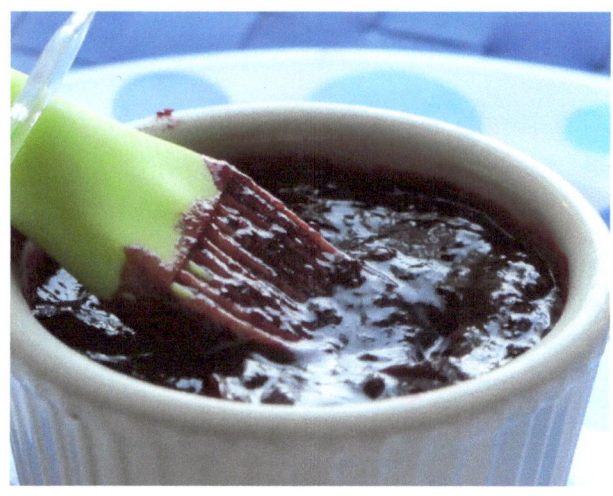

Nutrition Notes (per serving): Calories 23; Protein 0.2 g; Carbs 5 g; Fat 1 g; Sugar 4 g

Toppings

ALL-PURPOSE CRUMBLE TOPPING

The beauty of a crumble topping is its simplicity, but also its flexibility. It's about combining the butter-sugar-flour ratio to fit your fruit dish and your preferences. A typical sugar-butter-flour ratio for a crumble is 1:1:2, which results in a fairly crunchy topping. Although not exactly using this ratio, the version below is my favorite crumble recipe for blueberry desserts..

Makes about 2 cups (12 servings)

Ingredients

¾ cup (95 g) all-purpose flour

½ cup (100 g) brown sugar

2 tablespoons granulated sugar

¼ cup (23 g) rolled oats (not quick oats or steel cut oats)

Zest from ½ lemon

¾ teaspoon cinnamon

½ teaspoon ground nutmeg

¼ teaspoon kosher salt

½ cup (113 g) unsalted butter, cold

Directions

1. In a large bowl, mix together the flour, both sugars, oats, lemon zest, cinnamon, nutmeg and salt.
2. Cut the butter into small pieces and mix into the flour mixture with your hands or a pastry cutter or two forks until you have a coarse, pea-sized crumb. It's OK if small pieces of the butter are not thoroughly incorporated.
3. At this point you can refrigerate the mixture, covered, for 3 days or freeze in an airtight container for 3 months.

Substitutions & Additions

- Avoid instant oats as they will get mushy and avoid steel cut oats as they give a raw oat taste rather than the crunchy sweet taste.
- Add ¼ cup pecans or other nuts for more crunch.

Cooking Notes

- Crumble ingredients: Butter and sugar assist in browning and a crunchy texture. Too much butter however, can result in a watery texture. Too much sugar can result in burning if you are dealing with long cook times. More flour and oats will give you a sandy texture and will result in a crumble that is more firm than tender.
- Use cold butter and do not overmix for the best texture.
- Choose the right size of baking dish for desserts with fruit fillings. If you're anything like me you will want a bite of the crumble topping with each bite of fruit filling. If you use a dish that is too deep, you will get a lot of stewed fruit with a thin layer of crust on top. A 9" diameter skillet with a depth of 2" is perfect for me.

Nutrition Notes (per serving): Calories 145; Protein 1 g; Carbs 18 g; Fat 8 g; Sugar 11 g

STREUSEL TOPPING

This is my go-to streusel topping that results in a sweet crumb with plenty of crunch..

Makes 12 servings

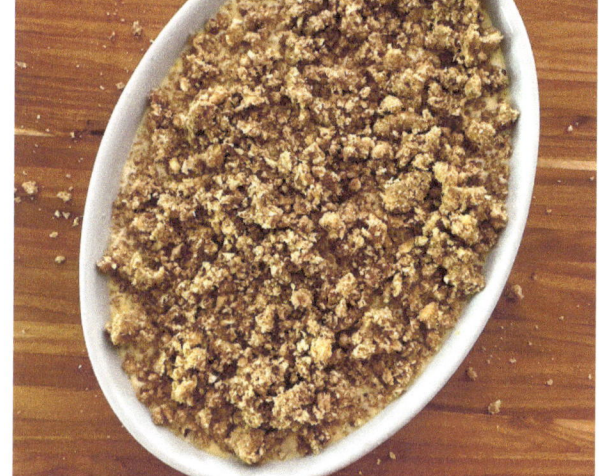

Ingredients

5 tablespoons (75 g) unsalted butter, melted and cooled a bit

¾ cups (94 g) all-purpose flour

½ cup (75 g) brown sugar

2 teaspoons cinnamon

¼ teaspoon salt

Directions

1. Soften the butter in a small bowl for 10-20 seconds in the microwave and let it cool for 2-3 minutes.
2. In a medium bowl, whisk together the flour, sugar, cinnamon and salt.
3. Add the cooled butter to the flour mixture and use a fork to stir it together until it forms uneven crumbs.
4. Set aside. Scatter streusel generously over muffins, pies, coffee cakes, etc., leaving a few open spaces for the filling or cake to peek out.
5. You can make the streusel the night before and keep it in the refrigerator. It will keep up to 3 days, covered, in the refrigerator or freeze for up to 3 months. Baked streusel can be stored in the refrigerator for up to 2 weeks, or frozen for up to 3 months.

Cooking Notes

- Additions that can be stirred into the flour/sugar mixture could include powdered ginger, cardamom, pumpkin spice or nutmeg.
- If you want to add nuts to the topping, finely chop about ⅓ cup and add to the flour/sugar mixture.
- Streusel can be used as a topping for most baked goods, but keep in mind that it tends to sink in thin batters, especially if you add nuts and heavier ingredients.

Nutrition Notes (per serving): Calories 105; Protein 1 g; Carbs 15 g; Fat 5 g; Sugar 9 g

Each recipe makes about 1 ½ cups (about 12 servings)

Vinegars/Vinaigrette

Fruit vinegars are similar to fruit shrub syrups, but with less sugar. They are simple to make and can be easily customized with infusions of spices or herbs. Fruit vinaigrettes, on the other hand, emulsify the fruit syrup mixture by the addition of oil (and often Dijon mustard). Vinaigrettes are savory and primarily used as salad dressings.

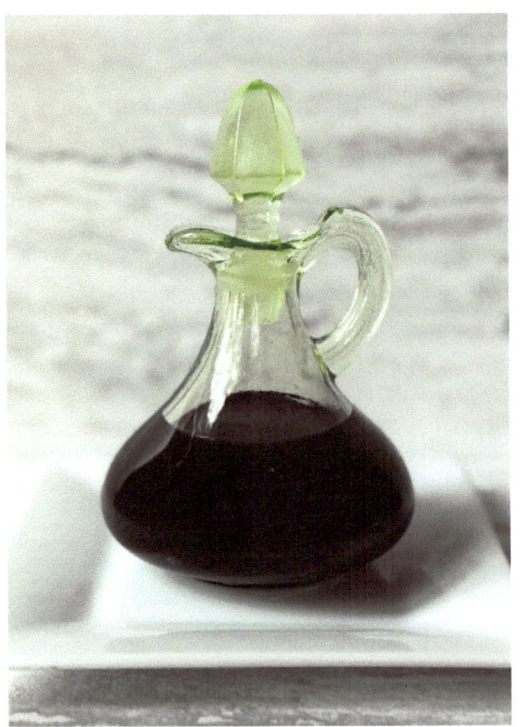

BLUEBERRY VINEGARS

Ingredients

2 cups (12 oz) fresh or frozen blueberries

2 cups (473 ml) white wine vinegar

2 tablespoons sugar

Directions

1. In a large non-reactive saucepan, crush the blueberries with a potato masher or back of a large spoon. Stir in vinegar and sugar; bring to a boil and stir until sugar dissolves.
2. Remove from heat and pour the blueberry mixture into a fine-mesh sieve that is placed over a large bowl. Allow the blueberry juices to strain into the bowl, leaving the solids behind in the sieve.
3. When completely drained, pour the vinegar into a glass bottle or jar and cover. Discard solids. The vinegar will last for several months, covered, in the refrigerator.

Substitutions & Additions

- Substitute champagne vinegar or white balsamic vinegar for the white wine vinegar. Avoid heavier, darker vinegars like red wine or red balsamic for optimal visual appeal.
- Blueberry vinegar can also be used to flavor drinks. Simply add 1-3 tablespoons to a 8 ounce glass of sparkling water for a spritzer, or add 1 oz (30 ml) to a martini or cocktail of your choice.
- Herbs and/or spices can be infused into the vinegar by adding them to the pan before boiling, turning off the heat and allowing them to sit in the mixture for 20 minutes before straining.

Nutrition Notes (per serving): Calories 29; Protein 0.2 g; Carbs 6 g; Fat 0.1 g; Sugar 4 g

BLUEBERRY VINAIGRETTE

Ingredients

1 cup (6 oz) frozen blueberries, thawed

¼ cup (59 ml) vinegar (balsamic, champagne, or white wine vinegar)

2-3 tablespoons sugar

1 tablespoon fresh lemon juice

2 teaspoons Dijon mustard

½ cup (118 ml) olive oil

Salt and pepper to taste

Directions

1. Mash the thawed blueberries with a potato masher in a bowl. You can use fresh blueberries, but they won't break down as readily.

2. Combine vinegar, sugar, lemon juice and Dijon mustard in a sealable container and shake or swirl to mix together.

3. Add the mashed blueberries and the olive oil to the container, secure the lid and shake well to blend. Refrigerate and shake again before using.

Substitutions & Additions

- If you have already made the basic blueberry vinegar in the recipe above, simply add ¼ cup of the blueberry vinegar, 2 teaspoons Dijon mustard, ½ cup (118 ml) of oil, ▢ teaspoon salt to a tightly sealed jar and shake vigorously to emulsify. Note: add a little sugar to the mix if your berries are tart.

- Olive oil is fine, but the blueberry flavor will be more dominant if you use a less robust oil like a canola oil.

Cooking Notes

- If your dressing is not properly emulsified, it may separate. Dijon mustard is an excellent emulsifier and helps create a stable vinaigrette that won't separate quickly.

- Another tip to prevent oil and vinegar separation is to slowly drizzle the oil into the vinegar mixture while whisking vigorously.

- You can customize the dressing with fresh herbs or garlic, but it will not last as long. Dressings with fresh ingredients (like garlic or herbs) will last about 3-5 days in the refrigerator. Dressings made with dried herbs and spices can last up to 14 days.

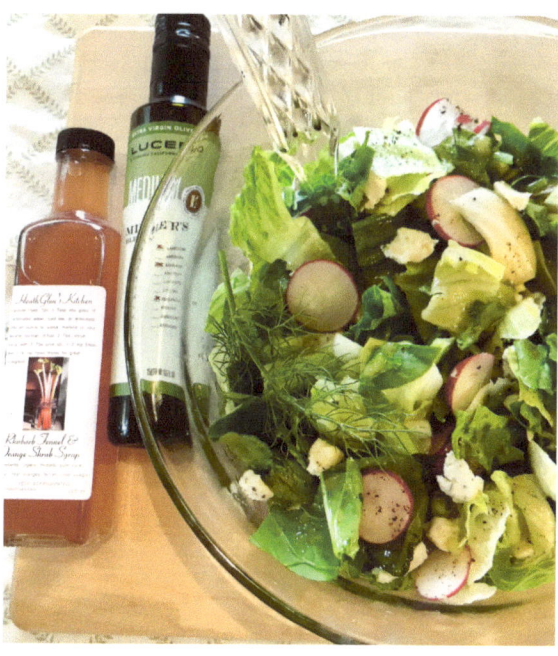

Nutrition Notes (per serving): Calories 96; Protein 0.1 g; Carbs 4 g; Fat 9 g; Sugar 3 g

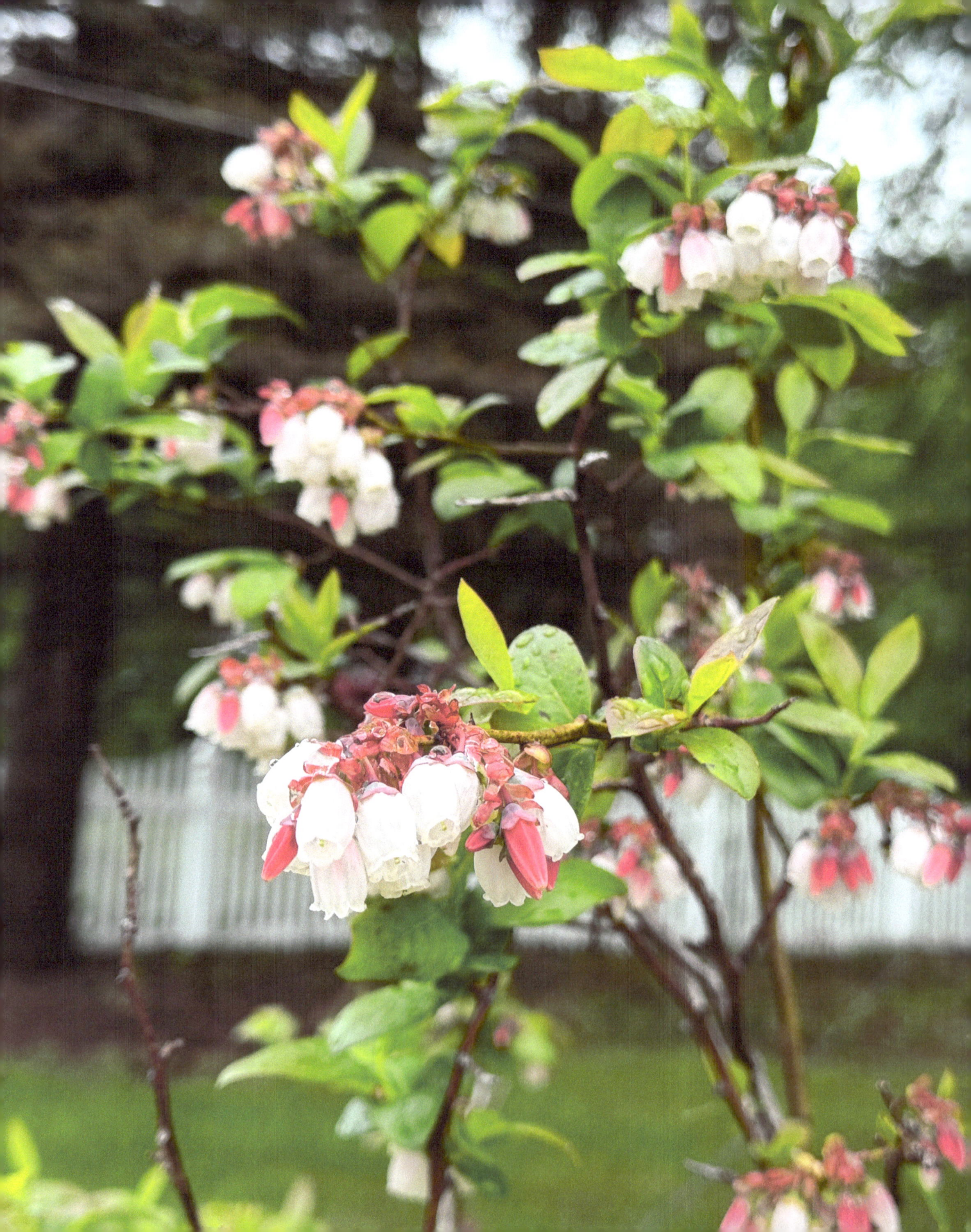

Part III
Helpful Resources

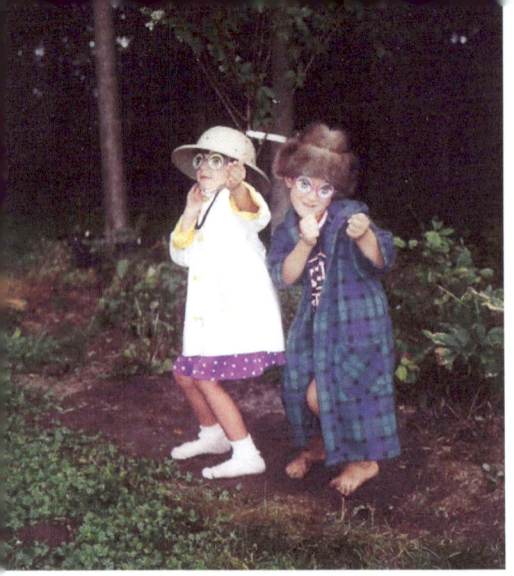
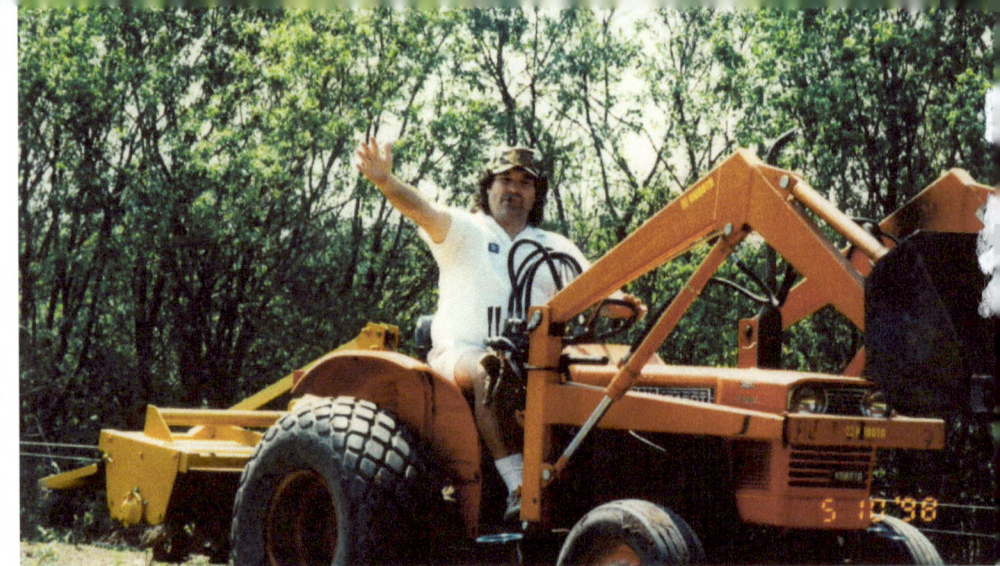
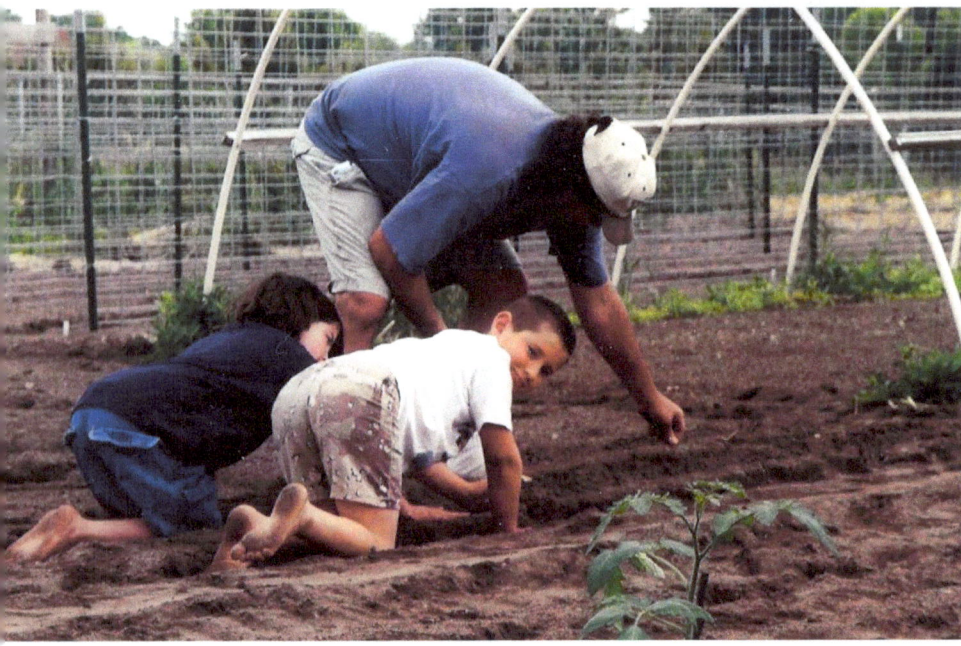
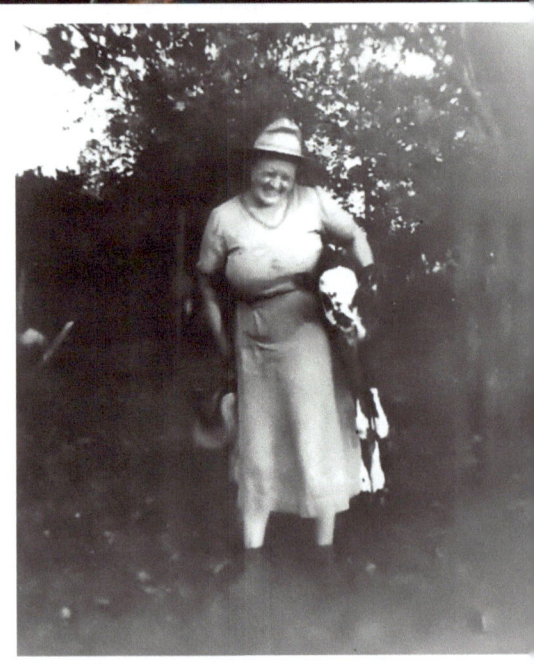
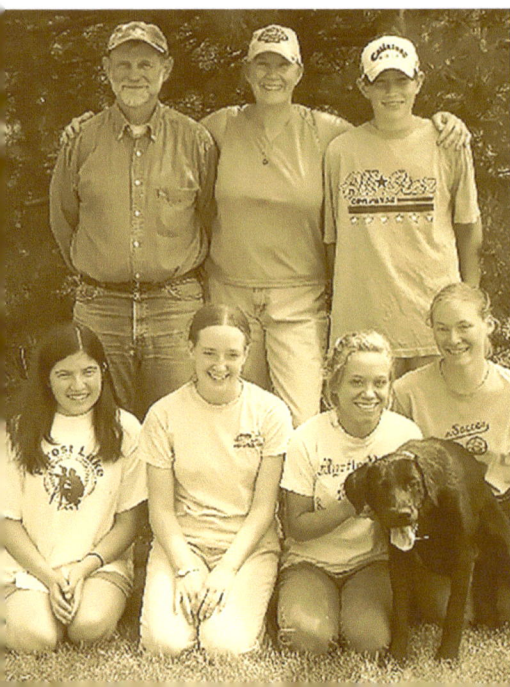
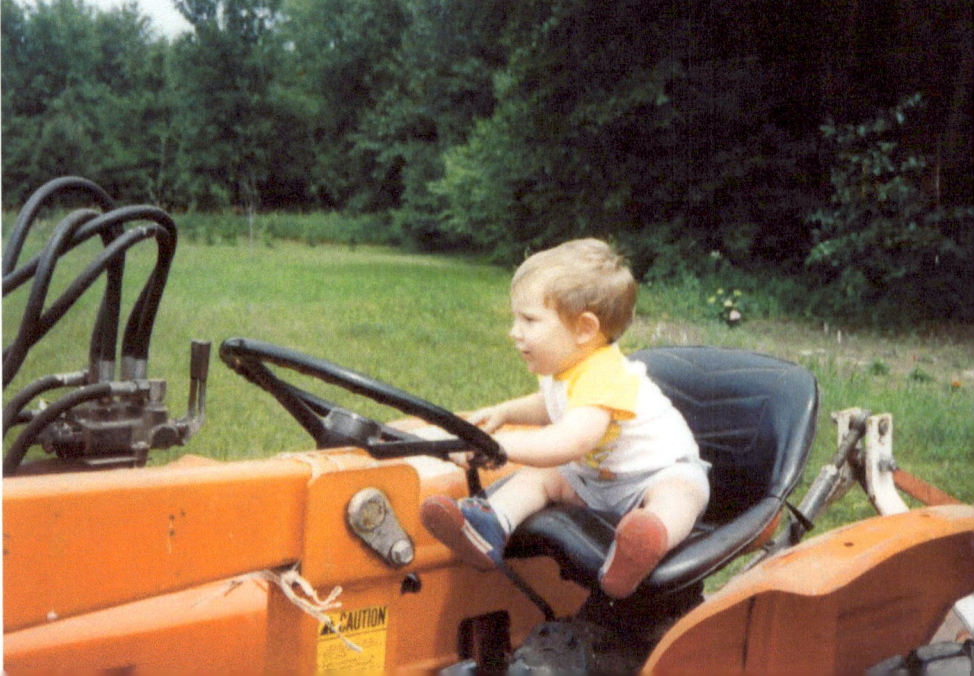

Helpful Resource Links

For Farm-to-Table recipes:
farmtojar.com

For new recipes, gardening tips, and health guides:
farmtojar.com/farm-to-jar-newletter

Guides & Tutorials for Growing Your Own Food:
farmtojar.com/category/grow-your-own-food/

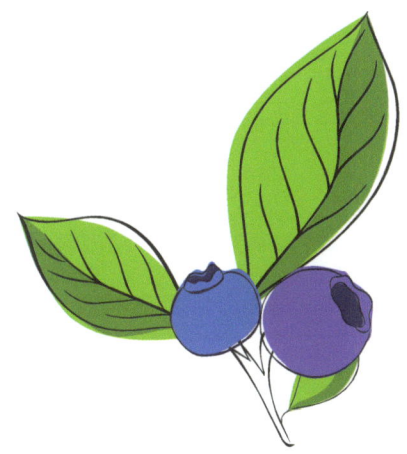

USEFUL EQUIVALENTS

The following charts are provided to help cooks who prefer using metric measures rather than US standard. All equivalents are approximate.

LIQUID INGREDIENTS BY VOLUME

- ¼ cup = 60 ml
- ⅓ cup = 80 ml
- ½ cup = 120 ml
- ⅔ cup = 160 ml
- ¾ cup = 180 ml
- ¾ cup = 180 ml
- 1 cup = 240 ml
- 1 ½ cup = 360 ml
- 2 cups = 460 ml
- 3 cups = 700 ml
- 4 cups = .95 liter

COOKING/OVEN TEMPERATURES

- Room temp = 68° F = 20°C
- Boil water = 212°F = 100°C
- Bake: 325°F = 160°C = Gas Mark 3
- Bake: 350°F = 180°C = Gas Mark 4
- Bake: 375°F = 190°C = Gas Mark 5
- Bake: 400°F = 200°C = Gas Mark 6
- Bake: 425°F = 220°C = Gas Mark 7
- Bake: 450°F = 230°C = Gas Mark 8
- Broil = Grill

DRY INGREDIENTS BY WEIGHT (BY SPECIFIC INGREDIENT)

- ⅛ cup = 18 g flour = 24 g sugar = 25 g butter
- ¼ cup = 35 g flour = 48 g sugar = 50 g butter
- ⅓ cup = 47 g flour = 63 g sugar - 67 g butter
- ½ cup = 70 g flour = 95 g sugar - 100 g butter
- 2/3 cup = 93 g flour = 125 g sugar = 133 g butter
- ¾ cup = 105 g flour = 143 g sugar = 150 g butter
- 1 cup = 140 g flour = 190 g sugar = 200 g butter

USEFUL EQUIVALENTS FOR BLUEBERRIES

- 1 cup = ½ pint = 6 oz
- 2 cups = 1 pint = 12 oz
- 1 pound = 3-3 ½ cups = 18-21 oz
- 1 quart = 4 cups = 24 oz = 1.5 lbs
- 1 cup = 65-75 blueberries = 148 - 190 g
- 1 cup @ 148 g = 84 calories

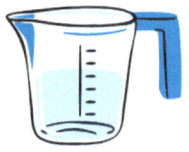
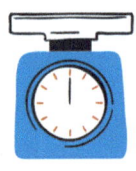
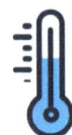
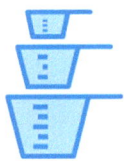

Index

A
Alcohol
  adding to drinks, 117-119
  used in cooking, 135

B
Bakeware, 9-11
Baking powder, 7
Baking soda, 7
Basil
  Basil Lemonade, 115
  Cornish Game Hens, 63
  Prosciutto Blueberry Pizza, 53
Blueberries
  about blueberries, 13-15
Breakfast Recipes, 20-47

C
Cake(s)
  Blackberry-Blueberry Poke Cake, 103-105
  Buckle Coffee Cake, 83
  Chocolate Sheet Cake, 99
  Cornbread Skillet Cake, 79
Cheese
  Blueberry Bacon Cheeseburger, 65
Cottage Cheese
  Blueberry Toast Variations, 25
Cream cheese
  Blueberry Cream Cheese Frosting, 99, 151
Goat Cheese
  Pizza with Prosciutto & Goat Cheese, 53
  With Pickled Blueberries, 131
Crustless Clafoutis, 71
Cheeseburger
(with Bacon & Blueberry BBQ Sauce), 65
Ricotta Cheese
  Breakfast Crepes, 45-47
  Fluffy Pancakes, 31
  Lemon Ricotta Cookies, 87
Children
  2-Ingredient Jam Tarts, 69
  Cooking for, 22, 27
  Farming with, introduction

Chocolate
  Chocolate Sheet Cake, 99
Clafoutis, 71
Cobbler
  Cornmeal Biscuit Blueberry Cobbler, 77
Cocktail(s)
  Blueberry Martini, 119
  Blueberry Mojito, 119
  using simple syrup, 129
Compote (see also sauces)
  All-Around Blueberry Compote, 152
  Blackberry-Blueberry Poke Cake, 103
  Blueberry Cream Cheese Frosting, 151
  Breakfast Crepes, 45-47
  Chocolate Sheet Cake, 99
  Fluffy Pancakes with Blueberry Topping, 31
  No-Churn Ice Cream Sandwiches, 93
Condiments
  Blueberry Bourbon BBQ Sauce, 135
  Blueberry Corn Salsa, 137
  Blueberry Salsa Macha, 133
  Blueberry Vinegar & Vinaigrette, 156-157
  Pickled Blueberries, 131
  Salsa Macha/Chile Oil, 133
Cookies
  Cookie sheets, 9-11
  Ice Cream Sandwiches, 93
  Lemon Ricotta Cookies, 87
  Oatmeal Cookies with Dried Blueberries, 85
Cornish Game Hens with Blueberry Cumberland Sauce, 63
Cornmeal
  Blueberry Cornmeal Spoonbread, 81
  Blueberry Pie with Cornmeal Crust, 95
  Blueberry Plum Galette, 89
  Cornmeal Pie Crust, 146
  Cornbread Skillet Cake, 79
  Cornmeal Biscuit Blueberry Cobbler, 77
Cream. heavy whipping cream
  Blackberry Blueberry Poke Cake, 103-105
  Blueberry Cornmeal Spoonbread, 81
  Blueberry Scones with Earl Grey Tea, 41

Breakfast crepes, 45-47
Buttercream Frosting, 150
Cornmeal Biscuit Blueberry Cobbler, 77
Crustless Clafoutis, 71
French Toast Casserole, 35
heavy cream substitutions, 6
Lemon Posset, 73
Semifreddo, 109

Crepes
  Breakfast Crepes. 45-47
  folding crepes, 47
  sauce for crepes, 152

Crostata
  Blueberry-Plum Galette, 89

Crumble
  Skillet Blueberry Crumble, 75
  All-Purpose Crumble Topping, 154

Crust(s)
  2-Ingredient Jam Tarts, 69
  Blueberry Pie with Cornmeal Crust, 95
  Blueberry-Plum Galette, 89
  Cornmeal Pie Crust, 146
  Easy Pizza with Prosciutto & Goat Cheese, 53
  Finnish Blueberry Pie, 97
  Galette/Crostata Crust, 147

Custard
  Crustless Blueberry Clafoutis, 71
  Finnish Blueberry Pie, 97
  Lemon Posset, 73

D
Decorating see frostings and fillings
Drinks. 113-125
  Basil Lemonade, 115
  Blueberry Mint Smoothie, 21
  Cocktails, 119
  Looseleaf Tea, 121
  Italian Sodas, 117
  Mexican Berry Atole, 125
  Raspado (Mexican Shaved Ice), 123

E
Earl Grey Tea (scones), 41
Easy Desserts, 67-89
English Summer Pudding, 111
Equipment, 9-11
  specialty bakeware, 9-10

F
Fillings
  2-Ingredient Jam Tarts, 69
  All-Around Blueberry Compote, 152
  Classic Blueberry Pie, 95
  Blueberry-Plum Galette, 89
  Breakfast Crepes with Ricotta Filling, 45-47
  Sour cream filling, Finnish Blueberry Pie, 97
  Skillet Blueberry Crumble, 75
  thickeners for, 6
Finnish Blueberry Pie, 97
Flour, about, 4
Foundational Recipes, 146-157
Frostings
  Blueberry Buttercream Frosting, 150
  Blueberry Cream Cheese Frosting, 151
Frozen
  using frozen blueberries, 6,13-15
  High-Protein Blueberry Mint Smoothie, 21

G
Galette
  Blueberry-Plum Galette, 89
  Galette/Crostata Dough, 147-148
Glazes
  Blueberry Glazed Baby Back Ribs, 61
Goat Cheese
  4 Blueberry Toast Variations, 25
  Pickled Blueberries with Goat Cheese, 131
  Pizza with Prosciutto and Goat Cheese, 53
Grunts, 95

H
Herbs (see specific herbs by name)

I
Ice cream
  No-Churn Ice Cream Sandwiches, 93
  Semifreddo: No-Churn Ice Cream Dessert, 109
Icing (see frostings)
Ingredients
  about, 4-7
Italian
  Italian Sodas, 117
  Italian Soda Syrup, 129
  Lemon Ricotta Cookies, 87

J

Jam
- 2- Ingredient Jam Tarts, 69
- 4 Blueberry Toast Variations, 25
- Blueberry Buttercream Frosting, 150
- Blueberry Lavender Merlot Jam, 143
- Blueberry Yogurt Breakfast Popsicles, 27
- Lemon Blueberry Souffle, 107

L

Lavender
- Culinary lavender, 6
- Blueberry Lavender Merlot Jam, 143
- Scones with Earl Grey Tea & Lavender, 41

Lemon
- Basil Lemonade, 115
- Blueberry Zucchini Bread with Lemon Icing, 29
- Lemon Blueberry Souffle, 107
- Lemon Ricotta Cookies, 87
- Lemon Posset, 73
- using with baking soda, 28

Lime
- Blueberry Ginger Lime Muffins, 37

M

Main Dishes (Savory), 49-65
Metric Equivalents, 162
Milk
- High Protein Smoothie, 21
- Overnight Steel Cut Oatmeal, 23
- substitutions, 4,23

Mint
- Blueberry Mint Smoothie, 21
- Blueberry Mojito, 119
- Looseleaf tea additions, 121

Muffins
- Bakery Style Blueberry Muffins, 39
- Blueberry Ginger Lime Muffins, 37
- muffin tins, 9-10

N

No-Churn Ice Cream Sandwiches, 93
No-Churn Semifreddo, 109
Nuts
- in crumble topping, 154-155

O

Oats
- instant vs rolled vs steel cut, 4,23
- Oatmeal Cookies with Dried Blueberries, 85
- Overnight Steel Cut Oatmeal, 23
- Skillet Blueberry Crumble, 75
- Streusel Topping, 155

Oven temperature
- metric to US conversions, 162

P

Pancakes (see also crepes)
- Dutch Baby: Oven Baked, 33
- Fluffy Pancakes with Blueberry Topping, 31
- Poffertjes (Dutch Fair Food), 101

Pans
- about baking pans, 9-11

Pantry
- useful pantry items, 4-7
- for storage, 139

Pickled Blueberries, 131

Pies and tarts
- baking dish sizes, 11
- Blueberry-Plum Galette, 89
- Classic Blueberry Pie, 95
- Cornmeal Pie Crust, 147
- Finnish Blueberry Pie, 97
- thickeners for pies and puddings, 6

Pistachios
- Semifreddo with Pistachio Crust, 109

Pizza
- Prosciutto, Goat Cheese & Blueberry Pizza, 53

Plum
- Blueberry Plum Galette, 89

Poffertjes (Dutch Fair Food), 101
Pork Chops with Blueberry BBQ Sauce, 59
Preserves
- Blueberry Bourbon BBQ Sauce, 135
- Blueberry Lavender Merlot Jam, 143
- Blueberry Vinegar, 156-157
- Dried Blueberries, 139
- Pickled Blueberries, 131
- Salsa Macha, 133
- Simple Syrups & Shrub Syrups, 117-119, 141

Puddings
  English Summer Pudding, 111
  Lemon Blueberry Souffle, 107
Pumpkin
  4-Ingredient Jam Tarts, 69
  Squash & Brown Rice Salad with Chipotle Dressing, 55
  Streusel Topping, 155

R
Ribs
  Blueberry Glazed Baby Back Ribs, 61
Ricotta
  Breakfast Crepes with Ricotta Filling, 45-47
  Fluffy Pancakes, 31
  Lemon Ricotta Blueberry Cookies, 87
  ricotta vs cream cheese vs sour cream, 7
Resources
  Helpful Resources, 161-162

S
Salad
  Chicken & Blueberry Dinner Salad, 51
  Salmon & Blueberry Corn Salsa, 57
Sauce(s)
  Blueberry BBQ Sauce, 153
  Blueberry Compote, 152
  Blueberry Cumberland Sauce, 63
Skillet(s)
  Blueberry BBQ Bacon Cheeseburger, 65
  Breakfast Crepes, 45-47
  Cornbread Skillet Cake, 79
  Dutch Baby (in a skillet), 33
  Pork Chops with Blueberry BBQ Sauce, 59
  Skillet Blueberry Crumble, 75
  useful bakeware, 9-11
Souffe
  Lemon Blueberry Souffle, 107
Syrup(s)
  Basic Blueberry Simple Syrup, 129
  Blueberry Shrub Syrup, 141

T
Tarts (see Pies)
Tea
  Scones with Earl Grey Tea & Lavender, 41
  Looseleaf Tea with Dried Blueberries, 121

Toast
  4 Blueberry Toast Variations, 25
  Make Ahead French Toast Casserole, 35
Toppings (see also Foundational Recipes)
  All-Purpose Crumble Topping, 154
  Streusel Topping, 155

V
Vegetarian
  Squash & Brown Rice Salad with Chipotle Dressing, 55
Vinegars & Vinaigrettes
  Blueberry Vinaigrette, 157
  Blueberry Vinegar, 156

W
Whipped Cream
  Blackberry-Blueberry Poke Cake Topping, 103-104
  Semifreddo Dessert, 109

Y
Yogurt
  Blueberry Yogurt Breakfast Popsicles, 27
  Semifreddo Dessert, 109
  yogurt vs sour cream vs ricotta, 7

Z
Zucchini
  Blueberry Zucchini Bread, 29

Acknowledgments

In 2024, I decided it was time to take stock of my 25 years of experience with food, health and farming, and share it in a series of books.

The natural place for me to start was to write about the four specialty crops that I grow (heirloom tomatoes, chile peppers, heirloom squash and blueberries).

My first book on how to grow heirloom tomatoes was a small planner called **The Tomato Workbook.** You can find this planner on my website, **farmtojar.com,** or order directly from Amazon.

This second book is a cookbook focused on blueberries, and I have big plans for many more. Always good to have big plans!

With this book, the most pleasant surprise was the support I received from the women in the Minnesota Chapter of Les Dames d'Escoffier, and from my farmers' market customers. They jumped right in and became recipe testers, which was invaluable.

I'd like to personally thank the recipe testers that joined me on this journey. They added needed clarity on directions that would help beginning cooks, as well as flavor or texture enhancements that just made the end result taste better. Thank you to:

Robin Asbell	Gloria Baldino
Janet Boyle	Janice Cole
Donna Hempstead	Cindy Jurgensen
Lesley Martin	Terri Michels
Kim Ode	Tesla Stainbrook
Kristine Vick	Lauren Voigt
Genie Zarling	

I am so grateful to work on projects that I love, with people that I enjoy and admire. If you are interested in being a recipe tester for the next cookbook, or just want to stay updated, visit farmtojar.com/farm-to-jar-newsletter/ and sign up for my weekly newsletter.

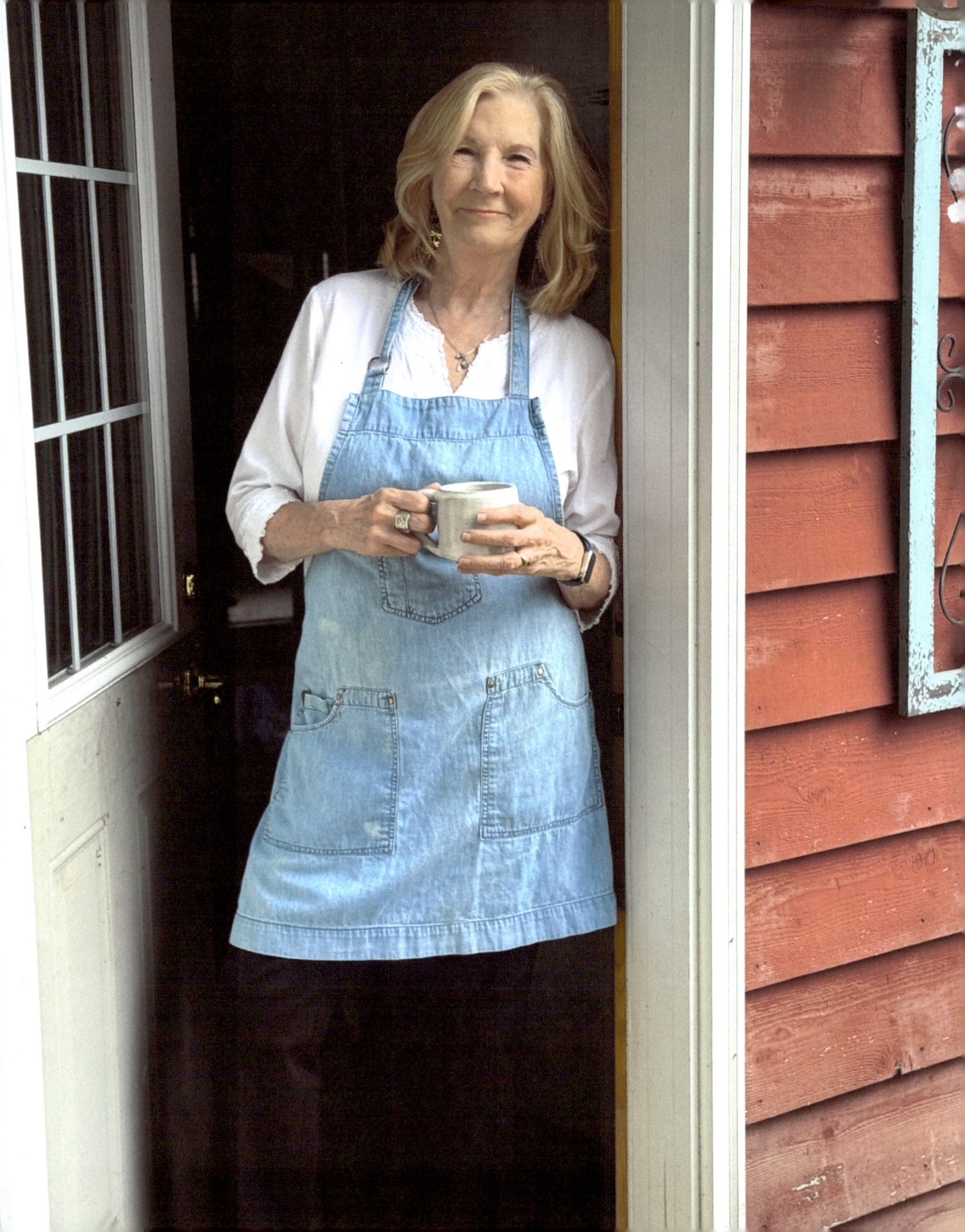

About the Author

Dorothy Stainbrook is a farmer, recipe developer, educator and founder of the recipe and gardening website called Farm to Jar. Her mission is to guide and inspire food lovers on the road to a joyful and healthy life through food.

Dorothy has been featured in *Sauveur* magazine, *Culture* magazine, *Urban Farm* magazine and *Wine Spectator*. She is also a proud 3-time Good Food Awards winner of her farm-fresh fruit preserves.

She is based in Forest Lake, Minnesota and lives with her tractor-waving husband, a smart wiry rescue dog, a goofy 100-pound lab, and a feline Queen Bee who supervises the whole team.

Find out more about Dorothy, her team, and her recipes at **farmtojar.com.**

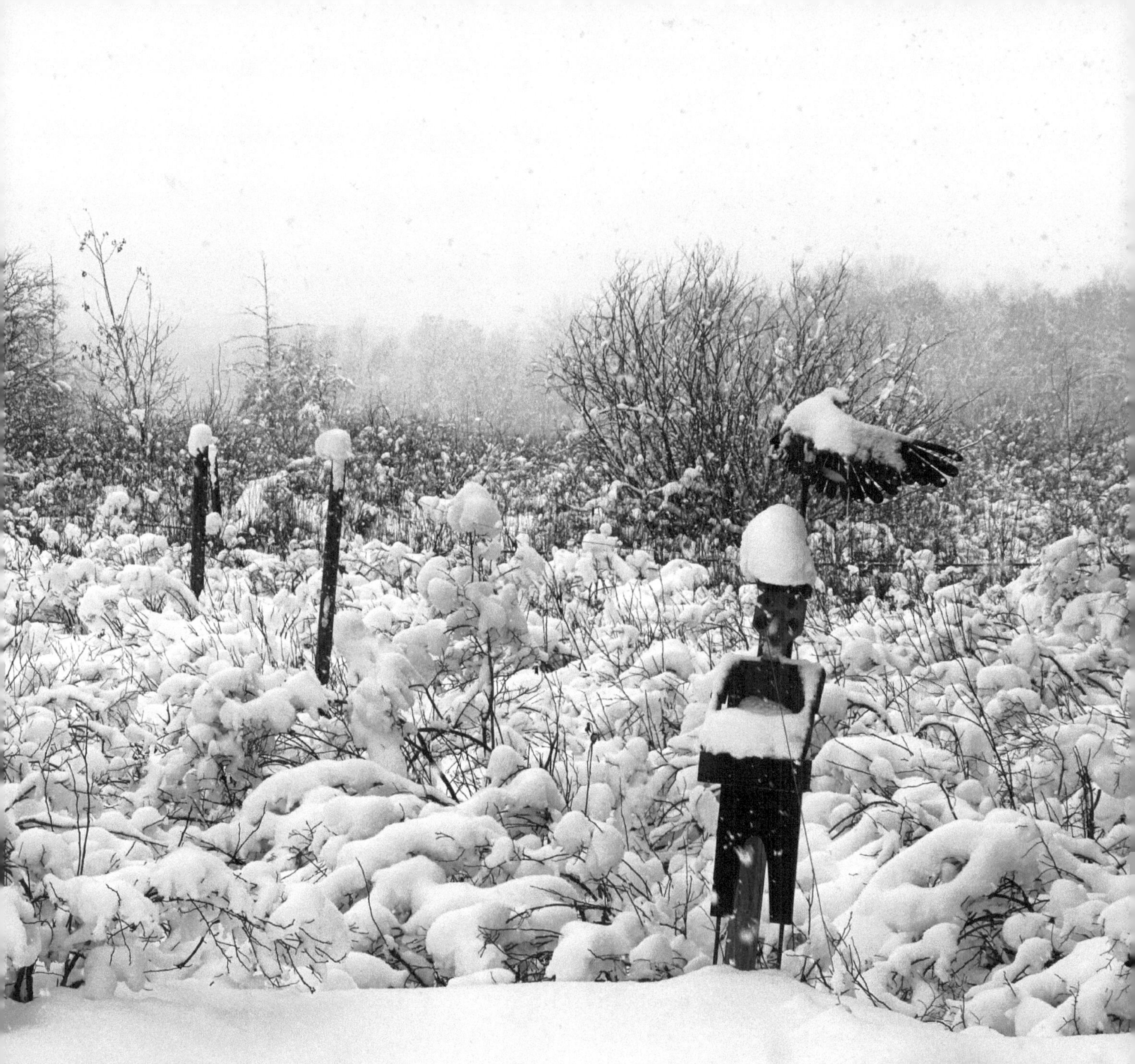

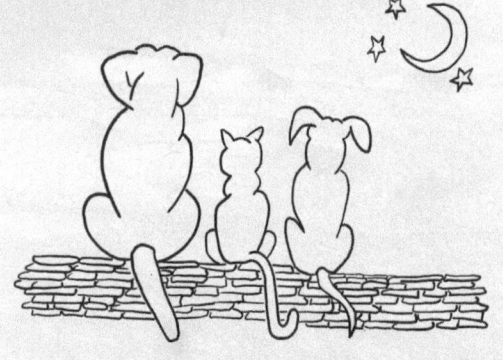

P.S. I truly hope you were inspired by some of these recipes, and I welcome your feedback. If you have any questions, don't hesitate to reach out by email **(dsheathglen@gmail.com).**